CHILD HEALTH NURSING REVIEW

ARCO NURSING REVIEW SERIES

CHILD HEALTH NURSING REVIEW

Luz Sobong Porter, B.S.N., M.S., Ph.D., R.N.
Associate Professor of Nursing
Department of Nursing
College of Human Development
Pennsylvania State University
University Park, Pennsylvania

Formerly Associate Professor and Director
Parent-Child Nursing Graduate Program
Division of Nursing Education
New York University
New York, New York

Associate Professor and Assistant Dean
College of Nursing
Silliman University
Dumaguete City, Philippines

**Arco Publishing Company, Inc.
New York**

Published by Arco Publishing Company, Inc.
219 Park Avenue South, New York, N.Y. 10003

Copyright © 1975 by Arco Publishing Company, Inc.

All rights reserved. No part of this book may be reproduced by any means, without permission in writing from the publisher, except by a reviewer who wishes to quote brief excerpts in connection with a review in a magazine or newspaper.
Library of Congress Catalog Card Number 73-94152
ISBN 0-668-03468-8
Printed in the United States of America

Editorial Advisory Board

Maurice H. Charlton, M.D.
Associate Professor of Neurology and Pediatrics
Director, EEG Laboratory
The University of Rochester
School of Medicine and Dentistry
and Strong Memorial Hospital
Rochester, New York

William M. Easson, M.D.
Professor and Head
Department of Psychiatry
Louisiana State University
School of Medicine
New Orleans, Louisiana

Menard M. Gertler, M.D.
Professor, Director Cardiovascular Research
Institute of Rehabilitation Medicine
New York University Medical Center
New York, New York

Martin I. Lorin, M.D.
Assistant Professor of Pediatrics
Director, Medical Education
Department of Pediatrics
College of Physicians and Surgeons
of Columbia University
New York, New York

Kenneth R. Niswander, M.D.
Professor and Chairman
Department of Obstetrics and Gynecology
University of California, Davis
School of Medicine
Davis, California

Charles Rob, M.D.
Professor and Chairman
Department of Surgery
The University of Rochester
School of Medicine and Dentistry
and Strong Memorial Hospital
Rochester, New York

For my Children
Carlene   Kevin   Brian
who are always a challenge to me

For my Parents
Jeremias E. and Expectacion C. Sobong
whose parental techniques I so adore

Contents

Preface		xi
References		xiii
Chapter I	TRENDS AND ISSUES IN HEALTH CARE FOR CHILDREN AND YOUTH	1
	A. Historical Perspectives	1
	B. Legislation	6
	C. Health Services and Organizations	8
	D. Education for Human Sexuality and Family Planning	12
	Answers and Explanations	19
Chapter II	THEORETICAL PERSPECTIVES OF HUMAN DEVELOPMENT	26
	A. Principles of Growth and Development	26
	B. Developmental Tasks and Milestones	29
	C. Developmental Correlates	35
	Answers and Explanations	42
Chapter III	HEALTH MAINTENANCE AND PROMOTION	49
	A. Physical Assessment	49
	B. Psychosocial Assessment	65
	C. Screening Tests	70
	D. Immunizations	79
	E. Nutrition	83
	F. Health Education and Counseling	88
	Answers and Explanations	92
Chapter IV	DEVELOPMENTAL PROBLEMS AND NURSING CARE	110
	A. Diarrhea	110

B.	Vomiting	113
C.	Cleft Lip and Palate	114
D.	Meningomyelocele and Hydrocephalus	115
E.	Cystic Fibrosis	116
F.	Diabetes Mellitus	118
G.	Autism	119
H.	Syndromes of Cerebral Dysfunction	122
I.	Convulsive Disorders	123
J.	Hyperkinetic Behavior Syndrome	127
K.	Mental Retardation	129
	Answers and Explanations	133

Chapter V   **SITUATIONAL PROBLEMS AND THEIR NURSING CARE**   140

A.	Hospitalization for Children	140
B.	The High-Risk Infant	148
C.	Accidents	151
D.	Burns	153
E.	Fractures	155
F.	Leukemia	156
G.	Rheumatic Fever	158
H.	Congenital Heart Diseases	160
I.	Respiratory Disorders	162
J.	Skin Conditions	164
K.	Other Situational Disorders	166
	Answers and Explanations	170

Chapter VI   **SOCIAL PROBLEMS**   179

A.	Child Abuse	179
B.	Drug Abuse	181
C.	Venereal Diseases	185
D.	Juvenile Delinquency	188
	Answers and Explanations	189

Preface

This book offers a comprehensive review of child health nursing, focusing on basic knowledge and understanding of the principles and skills underlying the family-centered care approach to children in health and in illness. It has been written for basic nursing students and graduate nurses to provide a concise and comprehensive treatment of the broad dimensions of pediatric nursing, identifying developmental milestones and basic pathophysiology of health deviations as well as critical details of nursing care. The content is organized focusing on the interrelationship of factors influencing health, illness, professional child health nursing practice, health maintenance, and the long term, acute and intensive care of children. The emphasis is within the context of an interdisciplinary approach to child health nursing. Supporting subjects such as nutrition, microbiology, pharmacology, anatomy and physiology are incorporated in the content.

The review questions are presented as situational problems, multiple-choice and matching questions divided into chapters by subject content. Each review item is individually referenced to current textbooks, monographs and journals. Corresponding answers and brief explanations are found at the conclusion of each chapter. The reference numbers and specific pages where the answers could be checked are indicated on the question pages. The question types are similar to those currently used on licensure examinations. A substantial portion of the content has been adapted from teacher-made tests on nursing of children derived from lectures, classroom discussions, and supplementary readings, and as such the content has been tested in a variety of classes.

Of particular interest to the reviewer is the historical perspective in Chapter One which sets the framework of this review book for identifying and developing trends and functions in family-centered child health nursing. Special attention is given to physical and psycho-social assessments of child health, clinical observations and the nursing process.

This book should be especially helpful to students of child health nursing and to graduate nurses needing a quick review of the basic knowledge and understanding pertinent to the care of children. Nursing graduates preparing for licensure examinations will find the book extremely useful. This book should also be helpful to technical nursing students as it provides different perspectives of pediatric nursing, presented in a highly organized manner. Vocational nursing students may find this book equally beneficial. Teachers in pediatric nursing will find supportive reference from this review book for quick content review and also for test construction.

The author wishes to acknowledge the valuable help of Linda Bellig, R.N., M.A. in preparing the materials on the high-risk infant, mental retardation, and the respiratory infections.

The secretarial assistance of Gary Pletsch and Loreto C. Sobong are highly appreciated. To those who have contributed directly or indirectly to this book by providing me a base of experience from which to write, I express my most humble gratitude.

Luz S. Porter, B.S.N., M.S., Ph.D., R.N.

References

Below is a numbered list of reference books pertaining to the material in the book.

On the last line of each test item, at the right hand side there appears a number combination that identifies the reference source and the page or pages where the information relating to the question and the correct answer may be found. The first number refers to the textbook in the list and the second number refers to the page of that textbook.

For example: (9:515) is a reference to the ninth book in the list, page 515 of Erickson's *Childhood and Society*.

1. Alexander, M. M., and M. S. Brown. *Pediatric Physical Diagnosis for Nurses*. New York: McGraw-Hill Book Company, 1974.
2. Anderson, B. A., M. E. Camacho, and J. Stark. *Pregnancy and Family Health*. Vol. I in *The Childbearing Family*. New York: McGraw-Hill Book Company, 1974.
3. Baldwin, A. *Theories of Child Development*. New York: John Wiley and Sons, Inc., 1968.
4. Broadribb, V. and C. Corliss. *Maternal-Child Nursing*. Philadelphia: J. B. Lippincott Company, 1973.
5. Bryan, D. S. *School Nursing in Transition*. St. Louis: The C. V. Mosby Company, 1973.
6. Child Study Association of America. *You, Your Child and Drugs*. New York: The Child Study Press, 1971.
7. Chin, P. *Child Health Maintenance*. St. Louis: The C. V. Mosby Company, 1974.
8. Chin, P., and C. J. Leitch. *Handbook for Nursing Assessment of the Child*. Salt Lake City: University of Utah, 1973.
9. Erickson, E. H. *Childhood and Society*. 2nd ed. New York: W. W. Norton and Company, 1963.
10. Green, M., and R. Haggerty. *Ambulatory Pediatrics*. Philadelphia: W. B. Saunders Company, 1968.
11. *Health Supervision of Young Children*. New York: American Public Health Association, 1965.
12. Helfer, R. E., and C. H. Kempe (eds). *The Battered Child*. Chicago: The University of Chicago Press, 1968.
13. Marlow, D. R. *Textbook of Pediatric Nursing*. 4th ed. Philadelphia: W. B. Saunders Company, 1973.
14. McCalister, D. V., V. Thiessen, and M. McDermott. *Readings in Family Planning*. St. Louis: The C. V. Mosby Company, 1973.
15. Mereness, D. *Essentials of Psychiatric Nursing*. St. Louis: The C. V. Mosby Company, 1970.
16. *Pediatric Annals*. Vol. 1, No. 3, Insight Publishing Company (December, 1972).
17. *Pediatric Annals*. Vol. 2, No. 2, Insight Publishing Company (February, 1973).
18. *Pediatric Annals*. Vol. 2, No. 5, Insight Publishing Company (May, 1973).
19. *Pediatric Annals*. Vol. 2, No. 9, Insight Publishing Company (September, 1973).
20. *Pediatric Annals*. Vol. 2, No. 10, Insight Publishing Company (October, 1973).
21. *Pediatric Annals*. Vol. 2, No. 11, Insight Publishing Company (November, 1973).
22. *Pediatric Annals*. Vol. 2, No. 12, Insight Publishing Company (December, 1973).
23. *Pediatric Annals*. Vol. 3, No. 1, Insight Publishing Company (January, 1974).
24. Redl, F., and D. Wineman. *Children Who Hate*. New York: The Free Press, 1951.
25. Rogers, M. E. *An Introduction to the Theoretical Basis of Nursing*. Philadelphia: F. A. Davis Company, 1970.
26. Taylor, D. L. (ed.). *Human Sexual Development—Perspectives in Sex Education*. Philadelphia: F. A. Davis Company, 1970.
27. Wallace, M. A. *Handbook of Child Nursing Care*. New York: John Wiley and Sons, 1971.
28. Wasserman, E., and L. Slobody. *Survey of Clinical Pediatrics*. 6th ed. New York: McGraw-Hill Book Company, 1974.
29. Wilson, C. (ed.). *School Health Services*. 2nd ed. N.E.A. and A.M.A., 1964.
30. Wing, L. *Autistic Children*. New York: Brunner/Mazel, 1972.

CHAPTER I

Trends and Issues in Health Care for Children and Youth

INTRODUCTION

The primary purpose of this chapter is to provide a framework within which you may gain an appreciation of the trends and issues in health care for children and youth and the challenges these pose.

The subject matter covers four broad areas, namely: historical perspectives, legislation, health services and organizations, and education for human sexuality and family planning. Multiple-choice and matching questions are utilized primarily to enable you to learn as many facts and principles as possible concerning the health care of children and youth. It is also projected that the use of these types of review questions will enable you to undergo an extensive self-evaluation of your current knowledge in the aforenoted areas of concern.

A. Historical Perspectives

Directions: For each of the following multiple choice questions, select the ONE most appropriate answer.

1. Which of the following statements does *not* accurately describe child care in primitive societies?
   A. primitive groups looked favorably on children who were strong and destroyed those who were not
   B. female babies were sometimes killed primarily for economic reasons
   C. birth of a deformed infant was always perceived as punishment for parents' previous transgressions
   D. isolated primitive groups had strong compassion for sick or weak children
   (13:3)

2. The first society that reared children to develop well-formed bodies was the
   A. Roman
   B. Greek
   C. Egyptian
   D. Chinese (13:2)

3. Which of the following peoples first exemplified the ideals of parenthood?
   A. Egyptians
   B. Romans
   C. Hebrews
   D. Greeks (13:4)

4. The philosophy of the sanctity of human life is a great influence of
   A. Mosaic Law
   B. the Hippocratic Oath
   C. Christianity
   D. Mohammedanism (13:4)

1

5. Which of the following individuals was the first to recommend that specific treatment for children's diseases must be differentiated from that given to adults?
   A. Celsus
   B. Hippocrates
   C. Confucius
   D. Maimonides (13:4)

6. The darkest period for child care in Great Britain and Western Europe was probably the beginning years of the
   A. Renaissance
   B. Industrial Revolution
   C. fifteenth century
   D. nineteenth century (13:4)

7. The first asylum for abandoned infants was founded in
   A. Italy
   B. France
   C. the United States
   D. Egypt (10:8)

8. About the middle of the seventeenth century, which of the following individuals organized a movement against the horrible practice of deforming infants and children for exhibition?
   A. Florence Nightingale
   B. Vincent de Paul
   C. George Armstrong
   D. Charles Dickens (10:8)

9. The first Children's Hospital in the United States was established in
   A. New York City
   B. Washington, D.C.
   C. Philadelphia
   D. Boston (10:9)

10. Which of the following factors has the *least* impact upon increasing incidence of infant mortality and morbidity?
    A. mother's age
    B. prematurity
    C. history of previous unfavorable outcome of pregnancy
    D. homogeneity of population (4:45-6)

11. Which statement below did *not* characterize child care in the United States by the middle of the nineteenth century?
    A. morbidity and mortality rates among infants and children were exceedingly high
    B. accidents in tenements and streets where children played were common
    C. child labor was never the problem in the United States that it was in Europe, nevertheless, children of the poor worked in stores and factories for inappropriately long hours
    D. most infants and young children were taken to boarding homes or baby farms (13:5)

12. The importance of the family was stressed in ancient Rome primarily because its function was to
    A. encourage children to learn as well as participate in outdoor activities
    B. transmit cultural heritage to future generations
    C. raise strong sons to become good warriors
    D. care for ill, helpless and infirm (13:4)

13. Which of the following ancient laws had a great influence on maternal and child care?
    A. Law of Hammurabi
    B. Mosaic Law
    C. Hippocratic Law
    D. Law of Maimonides (13:4)

14. Which peoples were the first to recognize the importance of cleanliness, nutrition, and communicable diseases and made efforts to control them?
    A. Hebrews
    B. Romans
    C. Greeks
    D. Egyptians (13:4)

15. Among the most important milestones in the progress toward improvement of child care in the United States was the establishment of the
    A. Children's Bureau and Office of Child Development

B. White House Conference on Children and Children's Bureau
C. World Health Organization and United Nations International Children's Emergency Fund
D. World Health Organization and White House Conferences on Children (13:8)

16. Which individual brought about sweeping changes in the care of children during the early years of the twentieth century?
    A. Florence Nightingale
    B. Lillian Wald
    C. Theodore Roosevelt
    D. Charles Dickens (13:8)

17. The first publication of the Children's Bureau was called
    A. *Prenatal Care*
    B. *Infant Care*
    C. *Children*
    D. *Children Today* (13:8)

18. The first world-wide health organization in history is the
    A. United Nations International Children's Emergency Fund
    B. International Red Cross
    C. World Health Organization
    D. International Organization for Health, Education and Welfare (13:9)

19. The organization mentioned in the previous question has its headquarters in
    A. New York, New York
    B. London, England
    C. Geneva, Switzerland
    D. Zurich, Switzerland (13:9)

20. The Halloween Trick or Treat effort traditionally participated in by American children is a means of raising money for the
    A. United Nations International Children's Emergency Fund
    B. World Health Organization
    C. International Red Cross
    D. International Organization for Health, Education and Welfare (13:9)

21. Which educational movement in the United States has led in compensating for the cultural deprivation of thousands of young children?
    A. Children and Youth Program
    B. Project Head Start
    C. Follow Through Program
    D. Maternity and Infant Care Program (13:12)

22. The care of children has changed dramatically during recent decades. All of the following are considered to be important factors, *except* the
    A. discovery of various immunization measures
    B. discovery of antibiotics
    C. utilization of public health measures and public education
    D. increasing use of wet nurses and increased mobility of families (13:14)

23. Much of the care of children in ancient civilization was done by
    A. wet nurses
    B. female members of the household
    C. religious leaders
    D. neighborhood ladies (13:3-5)

24. The following phenomena best describe the uprooting and movement of countless families in our present society, *except* the
    A. migration of rural families into large cities
    B. migration of middle-class to suburbs
    C. decrease in population of urban families in lower income groups
    D. increase in migration of families from other lands to U.S. shores (13:10)

25. Bronchiectasis is a highly prevalent disease among Alaskan children. This may be due to
    A. repeated inhalation of seal oil during feeding
    B. difficulty in providing preventive medical services
    C. repeated inhalation of coal dust
    D. difficulty in providing public health education (13:13)

26. Which one of the factors below was the major cause of serious intestinal disorders

among infants and children until the early decades of the twentieth century in the United States?
A. popular use of breastfeeding
B. ignorance concerning adequate nutrition and infant feeding
C. contaminated milk
D. increasing use of wet nurses (13:5)

27. Which of the following ancient laws provided that if a nurse allowed a suckling to die in her hands and substituted another, her breasts should be amputated?
A. Laws of the Twelve Tables
B. Salic Law
C. Theodosian Code
D. Code of Hammurabi (12:13-14)

28. All of the following individuals are famous for their leadership in raising public conscience awareness regarding the cruelty to children over the years, but which *one* earned the title of "Father of Nobody's Children"?
A. Thomas John Barnardo
B. Vincent Fontana
C. Charles Dickens
D. Samuel Halliday (12:13)

29. The American "Children's Charter" was adopted at the White House Conference on Child Health and Protection in
A. 1920
B. 1930
C. 1940
D. 1950 (12:15)

30. The first prenatal care to be offered by any group in America took place in 1901 initiated by the
A. Visiting Nurses Association of New York
B. Home Nursing Service of Philadelphia
C. Instructive Nursing Association of Boston
D. American Red Cross, Chapter of Los Angeles (25:1)

31. The rapid increase in scientific knowledge in growth and development of children and the etiology of illness have their greatest impact on the
A. medical profession
B. nursing profession
C. consumers of health services
D. all of the above (13:11)

32. An outstanding reason why cities tend to have high infant mortality rate is
A. increasing environmental pollution
B. sophisticated recording and reporting of vital statistics
C. migration to cities of many low-income families
D. increasing use of nurse midwives (10:83)

33. Which of the following statements is *not* a documented statement about infant mortality?
A. as of 1972, the United States lags behind twelve other nations in infant mortality rate
B. in 1920, the United States lagged behind five other nations in infant mortality rate
C. infant mortality rate among non-white population is two times more than white population
D. infant born in poor family has ⅔ chance that middle-class baby has of reaching first birthday (10:96,97)

34. The main objective of the founding of the Children's Aid Society of New York in 1853 was to
A. put public pressure against child abuse
B. move homeless children from streets into foster homes
C. raise funds for homeless children and indigent families
D. serve as children's advocate (13:all)

35. Which nation below was first to establish a full-fledged outpatient service as part of a children's hospital?
A. United States
B. Austria
C. England
D. Germany (10:11)

36. Which of the authors below wrote the book, *Textbook of Pediatric Nursing*?
    A. Dorothy Marlow
    B. Dorothy Johnson
    C. Violet Broadrib and Charlotte Corliss
    D. Florence Blake (13:all)

37. The publisher of the aforenoted book is
    A. C.V. Mosby Company
    B. J.B. Lippincott Company
    C. W.B. Saunders Company
    D. F.A. Davis Company (13:all)

38. A foremost leader in nursing education in the United States who is widely known for her strong views on nursing science is
    A. Jeanne Berthold
    B. Martha Rogers
    C. Louella Schlotfield
    D. Eleanor Lambertson (25:all)

39. An outstanding special problem affecting children of servicemen is
    A. separation
    B. accidents
    C. child abuse
    D. mobility (10:91,92)

40. The ambulatory services for children have been greatly enchanced by
    A. advances in diagnostic techniques
    B. availability of specific and rapidly acting drugs
    C. rising cost of in-patient care
    D. all of the above (10:35)

41. In the role of expanded pediatric nursing, the nurse
    A. performs physical examinations
    B. administers developmental tests
    C. manages diet, new foods and changes
    D. all of the above (13:14)

42. Which of the following countries have the lowest infant mortality rates in the world as recorded in the United Nations Population Census in 1965?
    A. Sweden and Norway
    B. Netherlands and Finland
    C. Switzerland and Denmark
    D. Netherlands and Sweden (10:96)

43. Comprehensive health care programs for children and youth can be enhanced by the following, *except*
    A. single entry centers for those who seek either health or social services
    B. use of nurse-midwives
    C. extended use of nurses in school health clinics, well-child conferences, and client counseling
    D. phasing out of existing health care delivery systems (13:74,75,76)

44. Which of the following is *not* an accurate statement about health and illness?
    A. what is health for one person at one time may be illness for another
    B. what is considered health varies widely between highly industrialized, technological societies and underdeveloped societies
    C. scientific and non-scientific orientations to health and illness are similar in their goals
    D. the belief that cause and treatment of illness are supernatural is characteristic of folk medicine (25:134-35)

45. Conceptualization of man's health-illness status as being determined by the interaction and integration of the internal environment of man himself and the external environment in which he lives and to which he relates is exemplified in which of the following theories?
    A. single-agent theories
    B. multiple-causation theories
    C. psycho-social theories
    D. ecological systems theories (25:135)

46. In the modern hospital, the nurse is an important component of the team. Her role includes
    A. giving direct care to children
    B. serving as a liaison between child and the physician
    C. serving as an interpreter to the parents
    D. all of the above (13:62,63)

47. Which of the following statements is true about the school nurse?
    A. she works as much in the community as in school as liaison and interpreter
    B. she is not a member of educational team for her concern focuses around health
    C. administers screening tests upon doctor's order
    D. she is primarily involved in improving family and community health as a whole (5:16,17)

48. According to Doris Bryan, the following are basic concepts in school health, *except*
    A. educational concept
    B. community concept
    C. space concept
    D. people concept (5:10)

49. An effective school health program is one that is dynamic and moving forward. Which school health concept depicts this framework?
    A. people concept
    B. educational concept
    C. space concept
    D. time concept (5:11)

50. Contributing factors to healthful school living include the following, *except*
    A. daily schedule of school activities best suited to maturity and capability of each child
    B. wholesome, clean and safe home environment
    C. planned food service program
    D. planned program taking into account health status of staff members involved in school (5:11)

51. Health education directed toward growth and development and toward affecting attitudes and habits is exemplified in the
    A. educational concept
    B. people concept
    C. community concept
    D. time concept (5:10)

52. The uniqueness in school health nursing, thus differentiating the nursing role from other school personnel, lies in the following attributes, *except*
    A. commitment to practice of health as quality of living
    B. application of nursing skills in dealings with individual health problems
    C. broad community health approach working through medium of educational institution
    D. strength of fragmented utilization of counseling, consultation, and teaching skills (5:2)

53. In terms of school nurse power, which one represents the highest level?
    A. school nurse coordinator
    B. school nursing educator
    C. consultant in school nursing
    D. school nurse practitioner (5:6)

54. The following are factors recognized as deterrents to school nursing practice as a specialty, *except*
    A. school nursing is stereotyped as a challenging and a complicated job
    B. school nurses believe "the old ways are good enough"
    C. school administrators often see nurse only as giving first aid
    D. health education is just off mainstream of American education (5:7)

55. Which of the following is *not* a component of the activities of the school nurse?
    A. health appraisal of all students
    B. health supervision in school hours
    C. health instruction
    D. diagnosis and prescription of treatments for infection (5:16-17)

B. Legislation

Directions: Match the following numbered items with the most appropriate lettered items.

56. Conference was focused only on concerns of young people, aged 14 to 24 years
57. Basic to many modern efforts in health care of children

58. Promoted opportunities for children and youth enhancing creative life in freedom and dignity
59. Establishment of first law for statewide care of handicapped children
60. Establishment of Children's Charter concerning health, education, welfare and protection
61. Establishment of Federal Department of Health, Education, and Welfare
62. White House Conference on Child Welfare Standards was convened

    A. Golden Anniversary White House Conference on Children and Youth
    B. 1919
    C. 1971 White House Conference on Youth
    D. 1930
    E. Social Security Act of 1935
    F. 1953   (13:6)

Directions: **For each of the following multiple choice questions, select the ONE most appropriate answer.**

63. The first Federal Child Labor Law was passed in
    A. 1917
    B. 1918
    C. 1919
    D. 1920   (13:5)

64. The *Declaration of the Rights of the Child* was approved by the
    A. 1950 White House Conference on Children and Youth
    B. 14th General Assembly of the United Nations
    C. Child Health Act of 1967
    D. Social Security Act of 1963   (13:6)

65. The *Pledge to Children* was adopted by the
    A. 14th General Assembly of the United Nations
    B. Golden Anniversary White House Conference on Children and Youth
    C. Child Health Act of 1967
    D. Midcentury White House Conference on Children and Youth   (13:6)

66. Which of the following agencies administers Project Head Start?
    A. Children's Bureau
    B. Bureau of Child Development Services
    C. Maternal and Child Health Bureau
    D. Office of Economic Opportunity   (10:75)

67. The first city in the United States to be in favor of tax-supported contraception for all people without regard to social or economic status is
    A. New York City
    B. Los Angeles
    C. Chicago
    D. San Francisco   (14:18)

68. Funds earmarked for family planning services within both maternal and child health, and foreign aid programs, were authorized by the United States Congress in
    A. 1968
    B. 1970
    C. 1967
    D. 1971   (14:20)

69. Which of the following organizations was the first to make policy statements on family planning?
    A. American Public Welfare Association
    B. Family Service Association
    C. American College of Obstetricians and Gynecologists
    D. American Public Health Association   (14:21)

70. Which of the following legislations provided the basic legislation and authorizations for maternal and child health, crippled children, and child welfare services?
    A. Title V of Social Security Act of 1935
    B. Title XIX of Social Security Act of 1965
    C. Social Security Act Amendments of 1963
    D. Social Security Act Amendments of 1965   (10:72)

71. Which of the following agencies serves as the epidemiologic surveillance branch of the United States Public Health Service?
    A. National Center for Health Statistics

B. National Institutes of Health
C. Communicable Disease Center in Atlanta, Georgia
D. Institute of Infectious Diseases
(10:74)

72. The Social Security Amendments of 1965 provide federal funds for
    A. training professional personnel for care of crippled children
    B. constructing facilities for care and treatment of mentally retarded children
    C. training teachers of handicapped children
    D. A and C (10:77)

73. The specific groups covered by Title XIX of the Social Security Act include
    A. children and youth who receive public assistance because of blindness and/or permanent and total disability
    B. all children and youth under twenty-one years of age who cannot qualify for public assistance, but whose families cannot afford to pay for all or part of the cost of medical care
    C. all children and youth under eighteen years of age whose families are indigent
    D. A and B (10:77)

74. Which of the following is *not* among the basic services mandatory for programs funded by Title XIX of the Social Security Act?
    A. in-patient hospital care
    B. physicians' services
    C. visiting nurse services
    D. x-ray and other laboratory services
    (10:77)

75. The United States Office of Education administers the following programs, *except*
    A. Project Head Start
    B. special classes for physically handicapped
    C. pre-school training programs
    D. school health (10:75,77)

76. In 1956, the United States Congress passed the Dependents' Medicare Act, which
    A. provides assistance with institutional care of handicapped dependents of service men
    B. provides financial support for transportation, training or medical care of handicapped children
    C. made available to dependents of military men certain medical services through civilian sources when not obtainable from military medical installations
    D. B and C (10:91)

77. The Army Health Nurse Program was instituted in
    A. 1942
    B. 1952
    C. 1945
    D. 1956 (10:90)

78. Which of the following services is a concern of the CHAP (Children Have a Potential) initiated by the United States Air Force in 1966?
    A. support to family life and counteraction of adverse influences resulting from husband or father being in a flying crew
    B. provision of advice on feeding and immunizations
    C. marshalling of available community resources to families with handicapped children
    D. provision of medical care to handicapped children (10:91)

C. Health Services and Organizations

Directions: For each of the following multiple choice questions, select the ONE most appropriate answer.

79. The national fact-gathering agency which serves as a goad to individual states to advance progress in child welfare legislation is the
    A. Bureau of Child Development Services
    B. Children's Bureau
    C. Children—Youth Service
    D. Maternal—Child Health Bureau
    (10:72)

80. Which of the following is *not* a main concern of the Children-Youth Projects?
    A. employment and training of community personnel for special recreational and counseling activities
    B. serving as a catalytic agent in strengthening community resources for disease prevention and treatment
    C. demonstrating a total approach to health needs of children in specified geographic area
    D. serving as an information source concerning drug abuse and teenage pregnancies (10:74)

81. Which of the following measures is likely to have the *least* influence in improving dental health services?
    A. curriculum changes to focus on preventive *rather* than restorative dentistry
    B. addition of fluoride to community water supplies
    C. securing community involvement and support
    D. training dental personnel to serve handicapped children (10:418)

82. In most school systems, education services for the homebound student are provided by the
    A. United Fund
    B. public school system
    C. P.T.A.
    D. Children's Bureau (10:74)

83. Which of the following is the health strategy identifying the purpose of the Health Maintenance Organizations?
    A. launch a national preventive health concept and improve efficiency of existing health services
    B. family planning and contraception control
    C. establish neighborhood health centers
    D. regionalization of health services in semi-rural areas and extension of clinic services in densely populated areas (10:73,76)

84. The agency that is charged with administering the Crippled Children's Program is the
    A. Office of Economic Opportunity
    B. Rehabilitation Services Administration
    C. Children's Bureau
    D. United States Public Health Service (10:74)

85. Which of the following agencies would be the appropriate one to refer to for assistance concerning a child with cystic fibrosis?
    A. Maternal—Infant Care Program
    B. Department of Health
    C. Rehabilitation Services Administration
    D. Children's Bureau (10:74)

86. A most recent and unique feature of ambulatory pediatric care in the United States is the
    A. trend for all health care of children to be entrusted to pediatricians
    B. emergence of group practice either limited to pediatric care or as a part of total family care
    C. trend toward fragmentation of health services to be provided by various specialists
    D. institutional fragmentation of preventive and curative ambulatory pediatric care (10:95)

87. Comprehensive health care reflects which of the following features?
    A. organized provision of health services to family groups
    B. use of health team concept with personal physician responsibility
    C. full spectrum of health services from prevention through rehabilitation
    D. all of the above (10:18)

88. The accelerated interest in delivery of health services is significantly influenced by the following factors, *except*
    A. national philosophic and budgetary commitment to belief that every child is entitled to health care of high quality
    B. large number of children receiving inadequate or no health supervision
    C. general recognition that hospitals and current medical programs have not been successful in providing adequate

health services to children of indigent families
D. apathy of community leaders toward role of hospital and other health agencies (10:34)

89. Which of the following statements is *not* generally true about health care received in out-patient departments?
A. health services are fragmented, episodic or crisis-oriented
B. attention is directed to total health needs of patient
C. quality of care does not approach in-patient standards
D. appraisals are quick and advice is hurried (10:34,35)

90. Which of the following principles would be the *least* effective for providing high quality health care?
A. regionalization of health services
B. comprehensiveness of care
C. continuity of care
D. compartmentalization of health care (10:36)

91. Which of the following approaches would deter the development and maintenance of quality health care?
A. utilization of allied health workers
B. availability of competent supervisors
C. deletion of out-patient departments in hospitals
D. in-service education among nonprofessional and professional staff (10:38)

92. In accordance with the organization of the United States Public Health Service, the Division of Nursing is under the auspices of the
A. Bureau of Health Manpower
B. Bureau of Health Services
C. National Institutes of Health
D. National Institute of Disease Prevention and Environmental Control (10:76)

Directions: Match the following numbered items with the most appropriate lettered items.

93. Plans for neighborhood health centers
94. Provides coordinated program of basic education, skill training and constructive work experience
95. Focuses on developmental activities and learning experiences for preschool children from low-income families
96. Provides opportunity for those eighteen and over to work with immigrant laborers, on Indian reservations, in slum areas, and in hospitals
97. Provides full or part-time work experience and training for youths sixteen through twenty-one years of age
98. Provides part-time employment of college students from low-income families

A. Project Head Start
B. Community Action Program
C. Vista Volunteers
D. Job Corps
E. Work-Study Program
F. Neighborhood Youth Corps (10:75)

Directions: For each of the following multiple choice questions, select the ONE most appropriate answer.

99. Which of the following statements is *not* true concerning organization of community health services for children, at state level?
A. each state has responsibility for hospitalization of mentally ill or mentally retarded
B. each state has an official agency responsible for operation of crippled children's agencies
C. each state has a welfare department responsible solely for child welfare services, such as adoptions and day-care services
D. each state has an education department responsible for such services as school lunch programs, special education, and, at times, school health programs (10:77,78)

100. The following services are *indirect* health services for mothers and children provided by local health agencies, *except*
A. surveillance of birth certificate for congenital malformations

Trends and Issues in Health Care 11

    B. provision of certain laboratory services such as virology and bacteriology
    C. health education of public
    D. well-child conferences   (10:78)

101. Which of the following is *not* an example of direct services for mothers and children provided by local health agencies?
    A. immunization
    B. diagnostic services for handicapped children
    C. public health nursing service
    D. none of the above   (10:78)

102. The public health nurse may perform the following activities, *except*
    A. screening of patients and taking routine measurements
    B. discussion of problems with mother and checking on child's development
    C. prescribing common medications
    D. giving immunization   (10:81)

103. Which of the following is a true statement about the hospital as a community health resource for children?
    A. role of hospital emergency clinic as a source of medical care for children is declining in importance
    B. as health problems of children have changed, hospital out-patient department is assuming a lesser role in health care of children
    C. considerable concern has been expressed about need to improve quality of hospital care given to children
    D. hospital pediatric out-patient department is primarily aimed at diagnosis, treatment and rehabilitation for children with long-term or handicapping conditions   (10:8)

104. The reasons why small communities in the United States reflect inadequate maternity and new-born care include the following, *except*
    A. shortage of high-quality staff
    B. geographic accessibility and transportation
    C. shortage of equipment and facilities in smaller hospitals
    D. nonavailability of medical specialists and resident staff   (10:83)

105. Which of the following statements is *not* an accurate statement of the special needs of children of migrant families?
    A. diarrhea and parasitic infections are common although immunization rate is high
    B. eye and ear infections are prevalent
    C. day care is usually not available to children although their mothers may be working in fields most of day
    D. children often go hungry, are undernourished and anemic   (10:83)

106. Which of the following is true about infant morbidity and mortality in the United States?
    A. in general, there is an inverse relation between per capita income and infant mortality
    B. the infant mortality rate in 1960 for nonwhites was higher than that for whites in all large cities
    C. in 1960 all of ten largest cities, except Los Angeles, had infant mortality rate higher than that for country as a whole
    D. all of the above   (10:83)

107. According to the United States Children's Bureau, the most prevalent chronic or handicapping conditions affecting children are
    A. hearing impairments
    B. eye conditions including refractive errors
    C. congenital heart diseases
    D. emotional disturbances   (10:85)

108. Recent trends that have facilitated increasingly comprehensive care for more handicapped children include the following *except*
    A. broadening of state's definition of handicapped child for eligibility of care
    B. developing evaluation, diagnosis and rehabilitation services for handicapped children on team basis
    C. incorporating children with chronic illness in organized home-care programs
    D. none of the above   (10:85)

109. Which of the following is a **unique feature** of ambulatory pediatrics in Eastern Europe?
    A. emergence of group practice either limited to pediatric care or as part of total family care
    B. availability of ambulatory preventive and curative health care of virtually all children delivered through pediatric specialists whose services are limited to a single group of families
    C. highly integrated and personalized system of care
    D. use of mobile units or payment to families for travel to health centers
    (10:95)

110. Which one statement below is *not* true about special problems affecting children of service men?
    A. mobility of family is a recognized feature of life in military services and its impact on children depends upon families degree of acceptance of move
    B. separation of father from family can be much more damaging than movement as far as child is concerned
    C. accidents and poisoning constitute same threat to military children as to civilian children
    D. more children of servicemen are abused and neglected than in civilian community
    (10:93)

111. The family health program is an example of which type of home care?
    A. community-based
    B. hospital-based
    C. medical-school based
    D. medical group practice
    (10:65)

112. The Coordinated Home-Care Program is aimed at
    A. coordinating home care in hospital neighborhood for patients who cannot afford a private physician
    B. encouraging early hospital discharge by arranging continuing supervision and rehabilitation at home
    C. dealing with all problems of child health and diseases outside hospital wards
    D. all of the above
    (10:64,65)

113. Which of the following objectives is *not* relevant to home care programs?
    A. to avoid hospitalizations, thereby decreasing cross-infection, emotional impact of mother-child separation
    B. to bring high quality "hospital" care into homes
    C. to seek alternatives to hospital care because of shortage of beds or nursing staff
    D. to study family in health and disease
    (10:65)

114. Which of the following characteristics of the rural health services in many developing countries are indeed relevant to current urban health programs in the United States?
    A. training and use of indigenous workers to improve communication between professional workers and consumers of health services
    B. use of mobile units or payment to families for travel to health centers
    C. training and use of subprofessional personnel to render simple therapeutic, as well as preventive, services in a clinic setting guided by standing orders
    D. all of the above
    (10:98,99)

D. Education for Human Sexuality and Family Planning

Directions: For each of the following multiple choice questions, select the ONE most appropriate answer.

115. The male reproductive organs include the following, *except* the
    A. gonads
    B. vas deferens
    C. fallopian tubes
    D. penis
    (26:5,6)

116. Spermatogenesis in humans begins at
    A. puberty
    B. latency
    C. adolescence
    D. adulthood
    (26:5)

117. Approximately how many sperm are expelled at any one ejaculation by fertile males?
    A. 100–300 million
    B. 200–500 million
    C. 600–800 million
    D. none of the above (26:5)

118. Which of the following is a fallacy?
    A. sperm can be transmitted to the female without ejaculation through lubricating fluid secreted by Cowper's glands
    B. sterility is related to virility
    C. removal of one ovary does not reduce sex drive or opportunity for parenthood
    D. tubal ligation does not reduce desire or orgasmic ability (26:5,6,7)

119. The partial skin covering of the vagina is called the
    A. prepuce
    B. external os
    C. hymen
    D. perineum (26:10)

120. The external genitalia of the female is otherwise called the
    A. vagina
    B. cervix
    C. clitoris
    D. vulva (26:10)

121. Orgasm is best defined as the
    A. summit of physical and emotional gratification in sexual activity
    B. act of ejaculation
    C. highly pleasurable, tension-relieving, seizure-like response to sexual activity
    D. A and C (26:11)

122. Which of the following is not true about human sexual behavior?
    A. male can impregnate at *almost* any time
    B. coitus is a means for producing orgasm in males and females
    C. orgasm can be achieved by female several times during single act of coitus
    D. ovaries *never* cease production of ova (26:8,11)

123. Twins can develop from the union of
    A. single egg and sperm or two eggs and two sperm
    B. single egg and sperm or two sperm and egg
    C. sperm and two eggs
    D. A and C (26:11)

124. Masturbation is best described as
    A. fondling of genitals either by self or others
    B. self-stimulation leading to sexual arousal and usually to climax
    C. self-stimulation leading to sexual arousal but short of ejaculation
    D. homosexual and heterosexual activities occurring before onset of puberty (26:19)

125. According to the psychoanalytic orientation, which of the following is *not* an expected manifestation of the oedipal conflict in boys?
    A. increased frequency of masturbation
    B. greater desire for physical contact with others, particularly members of the opposite sex
    C. diminished exhibitionistic tendencies
    D. intensified curiosity usually directed to mother (26:29,30)

126. Which of the following developmental tasks does *not* have to be accomplished as the adolescent moves toward adulthood?
    A. establishing heterosexual orientation
    B. achieving a masculine or feminine role
    C. getting started in an occupation
    D. selecting and preparing for an occupation (14:11)

127. An adolescent's emancipation from his parents is best assessed by the following criteria, *except*
    A. degree of his autonomy
    B. depth of his separatedness
    C. extent to which he trusts his own capacities
    D. degree of academic achievement (14:12)

128. While there is a real lack of systematic research concerning the sexual behavior of young people, the few studies conducted on college populations suggest that among females the trend is toward increase in
    A. consummated nonmarital and premarital sexual activity
    B. nonmarital and premarital sexual activity and involvement just short of intercourse
    C. use of IUCD's
    D. none of the above (14:188)

129. Natality and mortality data indicate that teen-age pregnancies run a greater risk than for older primiparas. The following are some of the documented risks, *except* increases in
    A. nutritional depletion
    B. number of school drop-outs without marketable skills
    C. percentage of forced early marriages
    D. drug abuse (28:29)

130. Which one factor below is the *most* important for the nurse to understand in order to be able to work with adolescents?
    A. concept of the "liberated" woman
    B. apparent decline in parental control
    C. cultural context within which a teenager struggles to find his identity
    D. developmental inconsistencies (14:188)

131. Which of the following data is the *least* important one in considering the health, educational, and social risks involved in school age pregnancy?
    A. about 50% of school age mothers will have subsequent unwanted pregnancies within two years following delivery of first child
    B. about 60% of those who have first babies at school age become welfare recipients
    C. one out of every six women in the United States gives birth within eight months following marriage
    D. school age mothers tend to have babies of low birth weight (14:53,58,59)

132. Which of the mechanisms below could enable a girl to find gratification and security in a feminine role?
    A. incorporating pattern of rival parent
    B. widening outside social contacts
    C. identifying with mother but repressing sexual aspects of identification
    D. all of the above (26:31,32,33)

133. The oedipal struggle normally occurs sometime between what period of development?
    A. first and fourth year
    B. third and sixth year
    C. second and fifth year
    D. fourth and seventh year (26:37)

134. The following changes are indicative signs of puberty, *except*
    A. accelerated growth of sex organs
    B. development of secondary sex characteristics
    C. nocturnal sex dreams
    D. occurrence of first ejaculation in boys and of menarche in girls (26:38)

135. Which set of behaviors below is *not* among the major types of directly sexual motoric activity that occur during adolescence and adulthood?
    A. tumescence, rock and roll dancing, tight fitting brassieres
    B. nocturnal sex dreams, homosexual contacts, orgasm
    C. masturbation, petting, coitus
    D. animal contacts, nocturnal emission, erotic stimulation of various parts of body (26:39,40)

136. Which of the following is a myth concerning the problem of illegitimacy in the United States?
    A. one out of every 12 children in the United States is born out of wedlock
    B. an estimated 50 to 75 percent of teen-age brides are pregnant at time of marriage
    C. more than 80 percent of females who give birth out of wedlock are teen-agers
    D. more than 40 percent of females who give birth out of wedlock are teen-agers (26:187)

137. Which of the following characteristics does not reflect a sex-linked recessive pattern of inheritance?
    A. affected persons are principally males
    B. sons of an affected male are normal, daughters carriers
    C. normal brothers of affected male cannot transmit disorder
    D. all female siblings of affected male will be carriers like their mother (10:190)

138. The genetic endowment of every individual consists of
    A. 23 paternal and 23 maternal chromosomes
    B. 24 paternal and 24 maternal chromosomes
    C. 46 pairs of homologous chromosomes
    D. 48 pairs of homologous chromosomes (10:189)

139. The unit genetic determinants are carried on the
    A. alleles
    B. locus
    C. chromosomes
    D. genes (10:189)

140. The desire for emotional satisfaction connected with wearing the apparel of the opposite sex reflects
    A. sex-role inversion
    B. transvestism
    C. homosexuality
    D. transexualism (26:79)

141. The phenomenon whereby a person of one biological sex learns to think, feel, and act like the opposite sex is called
    A. sex-role inversion
    B. transvestism
    C. homosexuality
    D. transexualism (26:79)

142. Which of the statements below does *not* accurately characterize deviations of human sexual development?
    A. although transvestism is a component of inversion, latter is not necessarily found in transvestites
    B. individuals who develop two sex roles are amnesic of existence of one role
    C. transexualism is primarily associated with men rather than women
    D. androgyny is associated with males who have female biological traits (26:80)

Directions: Match the following numbered items with the most appropriate lettered items.

143. Birth control method using abstinence from sexual intercourse during the woman's fertile period (2:50)
144. Cutting of vas deferens (2:61)
145. Round, rubber dome which is placed in the vagina to occlude the cervical os (2:55)
146. Contraceptive device fitted over the erect penis and prior to vaginal insertion (2:54)
147. Withdrawal of penis from the external female genitalia and vagina prior to ejaculation (2:54)
148. This device must be in place for at least six hours after intercourse (2:54)
149. An irreversible method of birth control (2:61)
150. Method is of very limited value since there is much difficulty in controlling actual time of ejaculation (2:54)
151. An example of the folk methods of birth control (2:54)
152. An effective device in preventing the spread of venereal disease during vaginal intercourse (2:54)

    A. Condom
    B. Coitus interruptus
    C. Rhythm
    D. Diaphragm
    E. Vasectomy

Directions: For each of the following multiple choice questions, select the ONE most appropriate answer.

153. Which of the following is a fact of human sexuality?
    A. females are inherently passive and males inherently active in sexual activity because of nature of sexual organs and coitus

B. penis envy leaves women with permanent scars of inferiority feelings and susceptibility to neurotic illness
C. clitoral and vaginal orgasms are separate, with latter being more mature, hence, more desirable
D. the lower one third of vagina is different morphologically from its remaining two thirds, hence, capable of accommodating any size penis
(26:196,197,198)

154. If any one of the four factors below is to be considered the end result of the development of a loving relationship, it should be
A. acceptance
B. understanding
C. sharing
D. esteem (26:308)

155. Which of the following responses should you make if a six-year-old girl asks you why she does not have a penis?
A. answer her question in a straightforward, simple way
B. refer question to her mother and/or teacher
C. show her pictures of nude boy and girl and focus attention on their genitalia
D. ask her to observe other girls and assure her that they, too, do not have a penis (26:34,35,36)

156. Tumescence refers to the
A. peak of sexual excitement
B. erection of the penis
C. penetration of ovum in decidual lining
D. period following sexual intercourse
(2:51)

157. The process that occurs when the ovum penetrates the decidua and becomes enclosed by this uterine lining is called
A. implantation
B. fertilization
C. conception
D. tumescence (2:51)

158. Another term for the above process is
A. dissemination
B. visceration
C. nidation
D. seeding (2:51)

159. Which of the criteria of conception control is met by the use of IUCD?
A. prevent union of sperm and ova
B. prevent ovulation
C. prevent permanent implantation
D. prevent release of estrogen (2:56)

160. The next most effective contraceptive method, and one that has been used for many years, is the
A. condom with spermicidal jellies
B. rhythm method
C. intrauterine device
D. diaphragm with spermicidal jellies
(14:35)

161. The contraceptives that offer greater effectiveness than any of the other methods are the
A. condoms with spermicidal jellies
B. oral contraceptives
C. intrauterine devices
D. diaphragms with spermicidal jellies
(14:31)

162. Which of the information below is true about the sequential form of oral contraceptives?
A. tablet containing only estrogen is taken for first 15 or 16 days of menstrual cycle
B. tablet containing only progestin is taken for first 15 or 16 days of menstrual cycle
C. tablet containing estrogen and progestin is taken for first 15 or 16 days of menstrual cycle
D. none of the above (14:31)

163. A tube that is put into each vas deferens with a valve to open or close the lumen is called
A. phaser
B. silastic implant
C. diaphragm
D. none of the above (2:57)

164. Which of the following is *not* true about contraceptives?
    A. the IUCD prevents ovulation from occurring
    B. the condom should be applied over the penis prior to vaginal insertion and should be removed immediately after ejaculation
    C. vaginal douche applied immediately following coitus is ineffective as contraceptive method
    D. coitus interruptus is of limited value as a contraceptive method since there is much difficulty in controlling actual time of ejaculation (2:54,56)

Directions: Match the following numbered items with the most appropriate lettered items.

165. Coitus interruptus (2:54)
166. Rhythm (2:55)
167. Oral contraceptives (2:55)
168. Tubal ligation (2:61)
169. Diaphragm with spermicides (2:55)
170. Condom (2:54)
171. Postcoital douche (2:55)

   A. prevents ovulation
   B. prevents union of ova and sperm
   C. prevents permanent implantation
   D. none of the above (2:54,55)

Directions: For each of the following multiple choice questions, select the ONE most appropriate answer.

172. The IUCD is usually inserted in what phase of the menstrual cycle?
    A. third or fourth day
    B. first or second day
    C. second or third day
    D. fourth or fifth day (2:59)

173. Which of the following may be experienced by the woman at the time of IUCD insertion?
    A. heavier than normal menstrual period
    B. cramps, bleeding or pain in back
    C. cramps, bleeding or pain in lower abdomen
    D. decreased menstrual flow (2:59)

174. An important instruction that a nurse should give to a woman with an IUCD is the necessity of
    A. medical check-up once in three months
    B. using supplementary spermicides
    C. checking for string or bead after each menstrual period
    D. checking for string or bead after each intercourse (2:60)

175. Which one of the following is *not* true about oral contraceptives?
    A. they are contraindicated in breast-feeding mothers
    B. withdrawal bleeding occurs within seventy-two hours after preparation is stopped
    C. they are prescribed either as combination pills or sequential pills
    D. if bleeding does not occur, pills should be restarted on tenth day after they had been stopped (2:56)

176. Concerning the effectiveness of contraceptives, which of the following methods is mostly ineffective?
    A. coitus interruptus
    B. vaginal douche
    C. spermicide foams
    D. prolonged lactation (14:31)

177. Which of the following is *not* a major side effect of oral contraceptives?
    A. edema and weight gain
    B. thrombophlebitis
    C. migraine headaches
    D. hypertension (14:32,33)

178. Women using oral contraceptives should be required to do which of the following at least annually?
    A. breast examinations
    B. cytological smear of cervix
    C. blood pressure determination
    D. all of the above (14:32)

179. There is no convincing evidence to date that the estrogen in contraceptive tablets causes cancer in humans. Which of the following research *findings* refute the aforenoted conclusion?

A. estrogen does induce epithelial change in breast tissue
B. cancer of the cervix has not resulted from use of oral contraceptives
C. estrogens are carcinogenic in several species of laboratory animals
D. none of the above (14:32,33)

180. To achieve its maximum effectiveness, the diaphragm must be applied as follows, *except*
A. put in place generally not more than an hour before coitus
B. left in place for approximately eight hours after intercourse
C. used with spermicides and left in place for approximately eight hours after intercourse
D. none of the above (14:35)

181. Indications for the use of family planning as a means of achieving optimum health conditions are reflected in the following research findings, *except*
A. reproduction occurring at ages 16 and younger, or 35 and older, is associated with the highest rate of perinatal death
B. combination of a very young mother, reproduction at short intervals, and high parity is especially associated with high morbidity and mortality
C. on a national basis, cases with no prenatal care had ten times the amount of overall mortality
D. history of abortion increases patient's overall mortality risk by 50%
(14:58,59)

Chapter I: Answers and Explanations

1. **D.**—There were isolated mothers, but not isolated primitive groups, who had strong compassion for the sick or weak children and did not necessarily live by the rules of the group.
2. **B.**—Physical beauty was considered very important to the early inhabitants of Greece.
3. **C.**—The Hebrews considered a large family as a sign of God's blessings upon the parents. The greatest disappointment a Hebrew woman could have was to be childless.
4. **C.**—Christianity was the first movement to teach the value of the child as an individual and not merely as son or daughter.
5. **A.**—Celsus was a Greek physician who lived in the first Christian century.
6. **B.**—During this period, children as young as six to twelve years of age worked in factories for ten or more hours a day.
7. **A.**—The asylum was founded in Milan, Italy by Archbishop Datheus.
8. **B.**—Vincent de Paul also established foundling institutions in France.
9. **C.**—The founding of the Children's Hospital in Philadelphia was considered to be the most important step ever taken towards the care of sick children.
10. **D.**—On the basis of several research studies, homogeneity of population is found to have the least influence upon infant mortality and morbidity rates.
11. **D.**—The practice of taking infants and young children to boarding homes or baby farms was common in Europe at that time, but not in the United States.
12. **C.**—The underlying motivation here was to produce good warriors who could serve the state.
13. **B.**—The Mosaic Law incorporated hygienic measures, nutrition, communicable diseases, and the like.
14. **A.**—The Hebrews, governed by the Mosaic Law, became very much oriented to a variety of health measures and made strong efforts to control communicable diseases.
15. **B.**—The White House Conferences on Children, since first established in 1909, have progressively led in advancing and safeguarding the well-being of children in all times. The Children's Bureau focuses on investigating and reporting upon all matters pertaining to the welfare of children across social classes.
16. **B.**—In 1903, Lillian Wald and Florence Kelly of the United States National Consumer's League triggered interest in the need for a federal organization that would be aimed at improving the conditions of children, and as a result, the Children's Bureau was established in 1912.
17. **A.**—This publication was introduced in 1913 followed by the publication of *Infant Care* in 1914. The Bureau's current official magazine is *Children Today,* formerly *Children*.
18. **C.**—The World Health Organization was established as a specialized agency of the United Nations.
19. **C.**—Whereas the headquarters of the United Nations is located in New York City, that of the World Health Organization is in Geneva.

20. **A.**—Money raised from the Halloween Trick or Treat effort is funneled to the United Nations International Children's Emergency Fund to help obtain medications and food for many ill and impoverished children throughout the world.
21. **B.**—The Project Head Start was developed to help culturally deprived children, as they have been found to do very poorly in schools.
22. **D.**—The use of wet nurses has decreased tremendously during recent years.
23. **B.**—Child care in ancient civilizations was primarily under the supervision of the women of the household. These women may have been aunts and grandmothers, as families were then of the extended type.
24. **C.**—There has been an increasing migration of the lower income groups to cities in recent years.
25. **A.**—Repeated inhalation of seal oil readily results in lipoid pneumonia and frequent lung infections.
26. **C.**—Dairies and stores which handled milk were not inspected then and milk was not pasturized. Contaminated milk was indeed the major cause of serious intestinal disorders.
27. **D.**—Similarly, the Theodosian Code prescribed a death penalty for infanticide.
28. **A.**—Thomas John Barnardo demonstrated a concerted effort in London, forcing upon public conscience the existence of gangs of homeless children. He succeeded in establishing a chain of homes and vocational schools for the homeless children.
29. **B.**—The Charter pledged to every child a home, love, security, and full time public welfare services for protection from abuse, neglect, exploitation or moral hazards.
30. **A.**—Social responsibility soon became evident in licensing laws for protection of the public.
31. **A.**—Primarily, society expects the medical profession to implement the aforenoted advances with appropriate action.
32. **C.**—It has been demonstrated in various research studies that low-income families have more problems in implementing effective public health education and promotional health measures than any other group.
33. **D.**—An infant born into a poor family has ½ the chance that a middle-class baby has of reaching his first birthday.
34. **B.**—At that time, homeless children were just wandering around the streets of New York.
35. **D.**—The Berlin Children's Clinic and Polyclinic in Germany was also the first one to offer clinical instruction for ambulatory pediatrics.
36. **A.**—On the other hand, Broadrib and Corliss coauthored the *Maternal-Child Nursing*.
37. **C.**—W. B. Saunders Company is the publisher of Marlow's *Textbook of Pediatric Nursing*.
38. **B.**—Rogers wrote the book, *Introduction to the Theoretical Basis of Nursing Science*.
39. **D.**—The *mobility* factor bears a significant impact upon the child's personality development.
40. **D.**—The aforenoted factors have tremendously reduced the necessity for hospitalization unless deemed necessary.
41. **D.**—The modern professional nurse functions as health educator, advisor, researcher, case finder and as a compassionate and skilled nurse of the sick.
42. **A.**—It is of special interest to note that the two countries are separating their preventive and curative services. One wonders whether their extremely low infant mortality rates are indeed a reflection of their small population, homogeneous national cultures, common values and/or tradition.
43. **D.**—Rather than phasing out the existing health care delivery system, its weaknesses should be eliminated and strengths further reinforced.
44. **D.**—Folk medicine is based on the assumption that the cause and treatment of illness are organic.
45. **D.**—The ecological systems theories are based on the premise that man and his environment are open systems and each is constantly changing and being changed by the other.
46. **D.**—It is thus important that the nurse's educational background be interdisciplinary to prepare her for the many roles she is to play in nursing practice.

Trends and Issues in Health Care

47. **A.**—The school nurse is a member of the educational team. Furthermore, she administers visual and screening tests even without doctor's orders.
48. **C.**—The other basic concept is the time concept.
49. **D.**—"It is a program of multiple health activities going on today, built on the programs of yesterday, and planning for tomorrow."
50. **B.**—The question asks for factors contributory to healthful school rather than home living.
51. **A.**—All activities, including health services, must be educational in nature.
52. **D.**—It is the strength of *combined* and *not* fragmented utilization of counseling, consultation, and teaching skills.
53. **C.**—A consultant in school nursing must have at least a master's degree and be responsible in all areas of school nursing.
54. **A.**—School nursing is stereotyped as an easy job and without challenge.
55. **D.**—A school nurse is not expected to diagnose and prescribe treatments for infections.
56. **C.**—The participants truly reflected the diversity of American youth.
57. **E.**—This has been amended several times, however.
58. **A.**—The event was held in 1960.
59. **B.**—It was also in 1919 that the White House Conference on Child Welfare Standards was held.
60. **D.**—The *Children's Charter* is one of the most important documents in the history of child care.
61. **F.**—This was an outstanding legislation.
62. **B.**—Regional conferences were subsequently held to promote advocacy for mothers and children.
63. **A.**—Nine months later, such laws were declared unconstitutional.
64. **B.**—A year later, a White House Conference was held to promote opportunities for children and youths to realize their potentials.
65. **D.**—The theme of the said conference was *A Fair Chance to Achieve a Healthy Personality*.
66. **D.**—The Project Head Start is aimed at preparing culturally deprived children for entry into kindergarten or the first grade.
67. **A.**—This event first took place in 1957.
68. **C.**—The importance of the population problem was concurrently emphasized by 30 constituents of the United Nations on Human Rights Day.
69. **D.**—The American Public Health Association made a policy statement in 1959 and another one in 1964.
70. **A.**—Title V of the Social Security Act of 1935, which is being administered by the Children's Bureau, provided the basic legislation and authorizations for the maternal and child health, crippled children and child welfare services.
71. **C.**—The United States Public Health Service also has special units working on accident prevention, dental health, heart disease, and the like.
72. **A.**—It also provides authorization for continuation of federal funds for statewide programs in mental retardation.
73. **D.**—The age limit is 21 years of age rather than 18.
74. **C.**—Visiting nurse service is a part, but not a mandatory basic service, of programs funded by Title XIX of the Social Security Act.
75. **A.**—Project Head Start is administered by the Office of Economic Opportunity.
76. **C.**—A and B are 1966 amendments.
77. **B.**—This legislation was primarily instituted to free the physician from tasks that only he could previously accomplish.
78. **C.**—The CHAP program compiles a listing of special community resources available for the handicapped child, and where and how to apply for these resources.
79. **B.**—The Children's Bureau is under the auspices of the Social and Rehabilitation Service.
80. **D.**—The problems of drug abuse and teenage pregnancies are primarily handled by centers or clinics so specified.
81. **B.**—The addition of fluoride to community water supplies is not really eliminating the basic problems underlying dental health services.

82. **A.**—The United Fund is primarily supported by nonprofit voluntary organizations.
83. **A.**—The Health Maintenance Organizations serve as cornerstones in reorganization of delivery of health services.
84. **B.**—Funds are used by the state governments to locate handicapped children, provide diagnostic services, and insure that each child receives medical care, hospitalization, and follow-up care.
85. **C.**—The agency provides services for long-term care.
86. **B.**—The practice is most recent and at this time provides services to relatively few children.
87. **D.**—This type of health care system certainly calls for an interdisciplinary health team.
88. **D.**—Community leaders are, on the contrary, increasingly interested in hospitals remaining responsible to current health needs and hospital practices being flexible, efficient and economical.
89. **B.**—Attention is often restricted to symptoms or signs of illness, and as such, medical care in out-patient departments is still primarily restricted to symptoms or signs of illness.
90. **D.**—Compartmentalization of health care represents an obsolete viewpoint. The health care system should be cognizant of the man-environment interrelation, which necessarily demands comprehensive health care services.
91. **C.**—The out-patient department is a very important aspect of hospital care and, as such, it should be further utilized rather than phased out.
92. **A.**—The Bureau in turn is under the auspices of the Office of the Surgeon General.
93. **B.**—The program is a means of providing actual health services for children and youth.
94. **D.**—The project is designed for youths aged 16 through 21 years who are lacking schooling and marketable skills.
95. **A.**—The Project Head Start programs are sponsored by local boards of education, church groups, or nonprofit organizations functioning under the Economic Opportunity Act.
96. **C.**—Work areas also include institutions for the mentally ill or intellectually retarded.
97. **D.**—Male enrollees are being provided with training in such occupations as automobile and appliance repair or work and building maintenance; female enrollees are being taught such services as household chores, graphic arts or child care.
98. **F.**—This program thus enables them to stay in or return to school or increase their employability.
99. **C.**—State welfare departments are now getting assigned responsibility for administration of medical care under Title XIX of the Social Security Act.
100. **D.**—The well-child conferences render direct services in supervising child health and diagnosing health deviations.
101. **D.**—The other choices represent direct health services.
102. **C.**—Prescription of drugs is not a part of nursing's functions.
103. **C.**—Indeed, there is a need to strengthen hospital pediatric out-patient departments as a main resource of child health care, as a model of comprehensive care, and as a principal training site for future pediatricians and nurse practitioners.
104. **B.**—Geographic accessibility and transportation remain a major problem in small communities.
105. **A.**—Immunization rate is low among children of migrant families; therefore, there is a prevalence of communicable diseases of childhood in this group.
106. **D.**—Infant and perinatal mortality illustrates the problem of the large cities.
107. **B.**—In 1970 there were 12,500,000 children and youths (5–17 years) who were reported suffering from eye conditions needing specialist care, including refractive errors.
108. **D.**—Other influencing factors are the establishment of combined centers for children with different types of handicaps and the inclusion of the care and rehabilitation of handicapped children in the training of health personnel.

109. **B.**—A somewhat similarly integrated and personalized system of care exists in Chile and is developing in other Latin American countries.
110. **D.**—There is no documentation for such statement. Service men are generally as interested in their children and make as good parents as their civilian counterparts.
111. **C.**—The program provides primary medical care for families of staff members and for the indigents in the neighborhood during health and illness.
112. **B.**—Encouraging early hospital discharge by arranging continuing supervision and rehabilitation at home is the goal of coordinated home care programs which are operating under a hospital or community based administration.
113. **A.**—The object is to avoid only *unnecessary* hospitalization.
114. **D.**—What may be found successful in other countries may not be necessarily so in the United States. This country shall have to seek its answers through problem-solving approaches drawing upon the experiences of other countries.
115. **C.**—The fallopian tubes are part of the female reproductive system.
116. **A.**—Production of sperm in humans is a continuous process rather than seasonal, as in some animals.
117. **B.**—Sterility is not necessarily related to virility.
118. **B.**—Low sperm count or immobile sperm is not necessarily associated with one's ability and desire to copulate.
119. **C.**—The hymen is usually broken by the first act of intercourse, but may also be broken through strenuous exercise, use of tampons or accidents.
120. **D.**—The vulva includes the mons pubis, labia majora, labia minora, clitoris and vestibule.
121. **D.**—Orgasm experienced by males and females is somewhat similar in nature; however, ejaculation occurs only in males.
122. **D.**—Cessation of ova production marks the menopausal period in females; nevertheless, the ovaries continue to secrete estrogen throughout the life of the female.
123. **A.**—Twin birth occurs in 1 out of 90 births.
124. **B.**—Homosexual and heterosexual activities may occur before or after puberty and a state of relaxation or satisfaction comparable to post-orgasmic state is sometimes achieved.
125. **C.**—There is a *predominance* of exhibitionistic tendencies in the boy during the oedipal period which accordingly offers him a reassurance that he still has a penis or serves to attract his mother's attention.
126. **C.**—Getting started in an occupation is a developmental task attained in early adulthood.
127. **D.**—Academic achievement is not a unique indication of the adolescent's emancipation from his parents.
128. **B.**—On the other hand, sexual behavior in males seems relatively unchanged over the years.
129. **D.**—Drug abuse is not specifically a part of teen-age pregnancy.
130. **C.**—Behavior is a personal manifestation or expression that is derived from two basic sources, namely (1) the many psychological, emotional and dispositional factors and (2) the power, influence, values and expectations that are initially external to the individual and are presented, assimilated and synthesized in a personal way. Thus, one must be aware of the context within which a teen-ager struggles to find his identity and come to terms with his new physical maturity.
131. **C.**—As long as the couple can take care of their baby adequately, it does not really matter that the baby was born within eight months following their marriage.
132. **D.**—Furthermore, the girl needs to divert her energies into nonsexual channels.
133. **B.**—Following the oedipal period, the child finally frees himself of the conflict sufficiently so that his energies can be diverted to other activities.
134. **C.**—Nocturnal sex dreams may occur during adolescence.
135. **A.**—The first set of behaviors, while always manifestly sexual, are only related to sexual activities; hence may be called proximal sexual motoric responses.

136. **C.**—Eighty percent is an exaggerated figure.
137. **D.**—Only half of the female siblings will be carriers and in turn they can expect half of their sons to be affected.
138. **A.**—This would mean 23 pairs of homologous chromosomes.
139. **C.**—The genes are the unit genetic determinants.
140. **B.**—Apart from their cross-sex apparel, transvestites may otherwise establish a heterosexual adjustment.
141. **A.**—It also involves the acceptance and adoption of the sex role of the other sex.
142. **B.**—Studies have demonstrated that they are usually aware of the existence of both roles.
143. **C.**—This method requires careful calculation of the fertile period from the menstrual cycle.
144. **E.**—Vasectomy is a relatively simple, hazard-free procedure usually carried out under local anesthesia.
145. **D.**—This device must be fitted to the user initially and refitted after pregnancy or after a weight loss or gain.
146. **A.**—The efficacy of the condom is questionable since it may leak, break, or come off during coitus.
147. **B.**—Coitus interruptus is of very limited value primarily because there are seminal secretions around the meatus prior to actual ejaculation.
148. **D.**—A diaphragm can be inserted any time before intercourse and to be extremely effective, it should not be removed or a vaginal douche taken for six to eight hours after the last coitus.
149. **E.**—Whenever a man chooses this method of contraception, he should be directed to seek medical advice and counseling to insure that he understands the implications of this particular method of birth control.
150. **B.**—Coitus interruptus could be a very frustrating experience to the couple.
151. **B.**—Other examples are post-coital douche and prolonged lactation.
152. **A.**—The condom is also considered to be more effective as a contraceptive device when used in conjunction with a spermicidal agent.
153. **D.**—The first three choices are some of the prevailing myths about human sexuality which, unfortunately, many people believe.
154. **C.**—Sharing is the tangible and experiential aspect of love, and enhances further understanding, acceptance and esteem of each other.
155. **A.**—It is best to handle such situations in a matter-of-fact manner.
156. **B.**—The penis must be in a tumescent state before it could penetrate into the vagina.
157. **A.**—Implantation is an important aspect of the process of becoming pregnant.
158. **C.**—The other aspect of conception is fertilization, a process preceding implantation.
159. **C.**—The IUCD is thought to cause the endometrium to secrete an enzyme preventing implantation.
160. **D.**—The spermicidal jelly will kill sperm that passes the barrier provided by the diaphragm.
161. **B.**—The use effectiveness rates for the pill average from 0.2 to 0.7 pregnancies per 100 women per year.
162. **A.**—This is followed by a tablet containing estrogen and progestin for the next 5 days followed by no medication for 7 to 8 days.
163. **A.**—This is one of the promising male contraceptive devices currently being tested.
164. **A.**—The IUCD prevents implantation rather than ovulation.
165. **D.**—As explained earlier, coitus interruptus as a contraceptive method is of very limited value.
166. **B.**—It must be remembered that a menstrual cycle can be affected by any kind of stress, hence the efficacy of the rhythm method is rather low.
167. **A.**—Oral contraceptives consequently prevent the union of ova and sperm as well as implantation.
168. **B.**—It is an irreversible method of birth control for women.
169. **B.**—The diaphragm bars the sperm from uniting with the ova and the spermicides serve to kill the sperm.
170. **B.**—It acts as a barrier to the union of sperm and ova but its efficacy is **doubtful**.

171. **D.**—This method has proven ineffective since it may propel the sperm closer to the external os.
172. **A.**—Bleeding may occur for a few days after insertion, and the woman may have a heavier than normal menstrual period.
173. **B.**—It is important that the client will have to be prepared for this experience.
174. **C.**—IUCD's have been known to be rejected by some women without their knowledge.
175. **D.**—The pill should be restarted on the *seventh* day.
176. **D.**—Prolonged lactation is mostly ineffective.
177. **A.**—The aforenoted signs will diminish or disappear within a few months of continued use; however, they are sufficient to cause some women to discontinue the use of oral contraceptives.
178. **D.**—Although to date no studies have demonstrated that estrogen can cause cancer in man, there is an absolute need to remain vigilant with the pill as any new drug.
179. **D.**—No studies to date have demonstrated that estrogen can cause cancer of the breast or any type of cancer in man.
180. **D.**—All the three precautionary measures increase the efficacy of the diaphragm.
181. **D.**—The overall mortality risk increases by *5%*.

CHAPTER II

Theoretical Perspectives of Human Development

INTRODUCTION

This chapter offers a brief, comprehensive review of basic theoretical considerations underlying one's understanding of human growth and development. It focuses on different concepts and principles as well as established facts and issues covering every stage of development from infancy through adolescence. As was done in the preceding chapter, the content is presented in multiple-choice and matching questions to enable you to do an extensive self-evaluation of your basic theoretical knowledge and expand further your knowledge and understanding of the developmental process in children and youth.

A. Principles of Growth and Development

Directions: For each of the following multiple choice questions, select the ONE most appropriate answer.

1. Factors influencing growth and development are reflected in the following phenomena, *except*
   A. females mature earlier than males
   B. greatest rates of growth are during fetal life, early school-age and adolescence.
   C. Down's syndrome is associated with short stature
   D. activity promotes growth   (28:2,3)

2. The only child is likely to develop more rapidly along intellectual lines than the average child because he
   A. gets the attention of the whole family
   B. is given strong encouragement to express himself
   C. is constantly with adults and is consequently mentally stimulated
   D. is apt to learn from uncles and aunts
   (13:29)

3. Which of the following is *not* an accurate statement of a principle of human growth and development?
   A. growth proceeds in biologically predetermined cycles throughout the life span
   B. all children go through a normal sequence of growth, but not at the same rate
   C. each child has his own unique genetic potentiality for growth which cannot be exceeded, but may be hampered at any stage
   D. individual pattern of growth and development is genetically determined
   (13:20,21,22)

4. A sharp deceleration of growth occurs from
   A. 2 years of age to pubescence
   B. 15 or 16 years of age to maturity
   C. 2 years of age to school age
   D. pubescence to 15 years of age   (28:3)

5. Which of the following phenomena is generally true about height and weight?
   a. greatest increase in height occurs during spring and least increase in fall

b. greatest increase in height occurs during fall and least increase in summer
c. weight gain is usually greatest in fall and least in spring
d. weight gain is usually greatest in winter and least in fall
   A. a and d
   B. b and c
   C. a and c
   D. b (28:3)

6. The progressive increase in skill and capacity of function best describes
   A. maturation
   B. development
   C. growth
   D. learning (13:21)

7. Euthenics is best defined as the science that deals with
   A. influences that improve hereditary qualities of race
   B. influences that improve acquired qualities of individuals and families
   C. measures to promote health for all age groups
   D. healthy uterine conditions for developing fetus (13:21)

8. The increase in physical size of the whole or any of its parts is generally referred to as
   A. growth
   B. development
   C. specialization
   D. maturation (13:21)

9. The production of a contour map of the hills and valleys of the whole human body employs the technique of
   A. physioprinting
   B. stereophotogrammetry
   C. grid-graphing
   D. sculpture (13:23)

10. The technique referred to in the preceding question is used for the following, except to
    A. serve as guide in tooth-straightening and denture-filling
    B. observe growth and development of premature infants
    C. measure physiologic differences among people
    D. study relation between mental retardation and body development (13:24)

11. Which of the following statements is a fallacy about developmental examination?
    A. tests of emotional and social development are less concrete than those dealing with physical or mental development
    B. developmental diagnosis is primarily aimed at assessing and interpreting maturity of nervous system
    C. developmental examinations tend to reflect all aspects of present observable behavior
    D. developmental examinations bear a high predictability in terms of later mental functioning (28:12)

12. If an individual is found to be in the 66th percentile in the height distribution of 100 ten-year-old girls, then
    A. 66 percent of comparable children should be of the same height as she
    B. 65 percent of comparable children should be shorter than she
    C. 65 percent of comparable children should be taller than she
    D. 35 percent of comparable children should be taller than she (28:4)

13. At about puberty, the trunk and extremities
    A. grow at different rates with trunk growing slightly faster than extremities
    B. grow at different rates with extremities growing markedly faster than trunk
    C. grow at equal rates
    D. none of above (28:5)

14. The constant interaction between the child and his family reflects the principle of
    A. undirectionality
    B. reciprocy
    C. helicy
    D. increased complexity (25:96,97)

15. The principle of helicy connotes that the
    A. life process evolves unidirectionally in sequential stages
    B. behavior of a person at any given time is a function of the state of that person and the environment at that point in time
    C. human field is interdependent with environmental field
    D. life process is an open system (25:99)

16. The cyclical nature of human behavior and of other universal phenomena embraces the principle of
    A. resonancy
    B. helicy
    C. synchrony
    D. reciprocy (25:101)

17. Eco-system is best defined as the
    A. total universe other than, and external to, system being considered
    B. set of combined units forming an integral or organized whole
    C. repeated set of relationships between man and environment
    D. total interacting system comprising living and nonliving entities and their environment (25:49)

18. Which one principle below does not reflect a homeodynamic system?
    A. reciprocy
    B. synchrony
    C. homeostasis
    D. resonancy (25:102)

19. The application of probability theory to nursing knowledge and nursing practice rests on *which* principle of human development?
    A. reciprocy
    B. helicy
    C. synchrony
    D. resonancy (25:99)

20. The potential for growth is greatest in
    A. early childhood
    B. late childhood
    C. early adolescence
    D. late adolescence (28:26)

21. In regard to the rate of physical development,
    A. boys tend to develop more rapidly than girls
    B. girls tend to develop more rapidly than boys
    C. there is no essential difference in the rate of development of boys and girls
    D. girls usually develop more rapidly than boys only for the first 1–2 years of pubescence (28:2)

22. Which of the following is the guiding principle about answering questions of children?
    A. tell child the truth to the best of your ability
    B. give information unemotionally and frankly
    C. outline facts briefly
    D. provide information, one fact at a time (13:520)

23. Any environmental change may have a traumatic effect on a child. Which of the following situations does *not* reflect the foregoing statement, in relation to the birth of a newborn brother?
    A. child makes derogatory remarks about newborn brother
    B. child kisses brother ending it with a bite
    C. child spends more time playing with neighborhood children
    D. child remains calm and plays alone in own bedroom (13:518)

24. When a child starts engaging in tasks in the real world, the nurse should recognize this change as the emergence of his sense of
    A. initiative
    B. industry
    C. intimacy
    D. autonomy (13:601)

25. Which of the following statements is true about relations with siblings?
    A. children in a large family tend to find sharing with outside group easier than does the only child

B. school children often prefer to be with their sibling rather than their friends
C. scholastic ability has little impact on sibling rivalry
D. the only child tends to cling a shorter time to his concept of being center of family's attention than child in a large family (13:604)

26. The eight-year-old child is best described as
    A. being modest about sexual matters and indulges in less sex play
    B. becoming oriented in time and space
    C. being in an age of broadening experiences and intellectual exploration
    D. entering the age when need for group activities is at its peak (13:609)

27. Which of the following statements is not true about learned behaviors?
    A. punishment weakens occurrence of behavior intended to be extinguished
    B. behavior that is rewarded will generally be strengthened
    C. purposeful ignoring should immediately follow behavior intended to be discontinued
    D. when desired behavior is being learned it should be reinforced every time it occurs (13:427,428)

28. "Gifted children" often begin to read
    A. before 5 years of age
    B. between 2 and 3 years of age
    C. at 3 years of age
    D. at 4 years of age (10:410)

29. To identify children as being especially gifted, intelligence testing should be administered as early as
    A. nursery school
    B. preschool
    C. early school
    D. middle school (10:410)

30. The basic principle in the management of the gifted child is to
    A. provide child access to materials which he can work with in his own projects
    B. arrange for special education
    C. help parents and others concerned keep in mind that a child with superior intelligence is still a child
    D. provide an enrichment program offering him special tasks, challenges and projects (10:411)

B. Developmental Tasks and Milestones

Directions: For each of the following multiple choice questions, select the ONE most appropriate answer.

31. Learning to relate oneself emotionally to parents, siblings, and other people is expected to take place in
    A. infancy
    B. early childhood
    C. middle childhood
    D. A and B (28:21,22)

32. In toilet training, an automatic function is placed under voluntary control through
    A. conditioning and maturation
    B. trial and error
    C. structuring and reinforcement
    D. experience and learning (28:20)

33. Which of the following developmental tasks is generally characteristic of eight-year-old children?
    A. change of attitude toward sex
    B. emotional outbursts of anger and frustration against parents followed by feelings of remorse and anxiety
    C. segregation of sexes important in choice of playmates and groups
    D. feelings of strength and self-sufficiency (28:22)

34. Which of the following characteristics, if seen in the adolescent male, can be considered to be fairly reliable indicators of his future sexual orientation?
    a. either aggressiveness or passivity
    b. either bluntness or sensitivity
    c. either self-assertiveness or reticence
    d. either a preference for outdoor activities or a preference for more sedentary activities

e. either stoicism or emotionality
A. b and e
B. a and c
C. d only
D. none of the above (13:686,687)

35. Sporadic homosexual experiences during adolescent years
A. may or may not predicate adult homosexual orientation
B. probably indicate latent homosexual tendencies
C. probably indicate overt homosexual tendencies
D. are rare (26:221)

36. The problem of establishing a sense of identity often is intensified if
a. one is of a minority group
b. the peer group is used for support and guidance
c. family relationships did not foster self-esteem
d. the adolescent begins to separate himself from his family tree
A. a and b
B. a and c
C. b and d
D. c and d (9:262)

37. If an adolescent shows a consistent way of acting in certain situations, it is most likely that he is evidencing
A. immature, stereotyped behavior
B. inability to be flexible
C. integration of personality
D. inability to problem solve (28:27)

38. Usually, dependence upon the peer group
a. becomes more evident during adolescent years than in earlier childhood
b. becomes less evident during adolescent years than in earlier childhood
c. indicates an emotionally unstable adolescent
d. should be discouraged if possible
A. a only
B. b and d
C. a and c
D. b and c (9:262)

39. Erickson postulates that the critical task in late childhood is the development of a sense of
A. autonomy
B. independence
C. industry
D. initiative (9:258)

40. Which of the following does *not* reflect egocentric thinking in a child?
A. he perceives consciousness as present only in animals
B. he cannot differentiate between the word and thing that the word names
C. he views dreams as coming from outside and taking place in the room
D. he regards everything that moves as alive (3:244,245)

41. A three-year-old child talking to himself as though he were thinking out loud is displaying a behavior that is
A. advanced for his age
B. retarded for his age
C. expected of his age
D. questionable (13:532)

42. A child who justifies his position at any price regardless of the reality of the situation is operating on the
A. preoperational stage
B. parataxic stage
C. concrete stage
D. syntaxic stage (3:192,243)

43. Which of the following behaviors is *not* indicative of a child's readiness for the transition period from home to school?
A. moves freely in pursuit of a wide range of goals
B. relates himself to others
C. imagines himself in many roles
D. none of these (9:255)

44. Which of the following is *not* likely to develop inferiority feelings in children?
A. limit setting and encouragement
B. insufficient solution of Oedipal conflict
C. poor teachers with whom to identify
D. emphasis on self-restraint and obedience to authority (9:259,260)

Theoretical Perspectives 31

45. Which of the following tells you that the child has attained the capacity to order and relate experiences to an organized whole?
   A. adds, subtracts, multiplies and divides
   B. visualizes sections and their displacement
   C. enjoys playing with puzzles
   D. all of these (3:249,250,251)

46. As the adolescent moves toward adulthood, he must essentially accomplish the following developmental tasks, *except*
   A. establish his heterosexual identity
   B. choose a vocation
   C. commit himself to responsible citizenship
   D. get started in an occupation (28:27)

Directions: Match the following numbered items with the most appropriate lettered items.

47. Preparing for marriage and family life (13:693)
48. Developing sense of trust (13:296)
49. Developing concepts necessary for everyday living (13:603)
50. Achieving one's physique and using the body effectively (13:692,693)
51. Learning sex differences and sexual morality (13:521)
52. Developing conscience, morality and a scale of values (13:520,521,522)

   A. Infancy
   B. Early childhood
   C. Middle childhood
   D. Adolescence

Directions: For each of the following multiple choice questions, select the ONE most appropriate answer.

53. A child is said to be operating on the reality principle if he demonstrates which of the following behaviors?
   A. delays gratification and tolerates unpleasant sensations for some future gratification
   B. identifies with another person
   C. questions about his dream
   D. prefaces all his responses with "no" (3:317)

54. The child learns about the limitations his environment sets through
   A. problem-solving
   B. reality testing
   C. trial and error
   D. continuous exposure (13:520)

55. Freud hypothesized that manifest dream content is
   A. unconscious thought
   B. disguised dream content
   C. always remembered upon awakening
   D. subconscious thought (3:325,326)

56. Freud also hypothesized that daydreams of childhood
   A. take the form of hallucinatory experience
   B. are meaningless and disguised
   C. are for purposes of wish fulfillment
   D. are used by children for complete id gratification (3:351,352)

57. After a child has learned to control his bowel function and uses it as a weapon to get back at his mother by defecating in an inappropriate place, he is said to be in the
   A. anal erotic stage
   B. anal retentive stage
   C. anal sadistic stage
   D. anal expulsive stage (9:81,82)

58. Which of the following is *not* associated with the phallic stage?
   A. increased frequency of masturbation
   B. predominance of exhibitionistic tendencies
   C. greater desire for physical contact with others
   D. tendency for boy to keep away from father (26:29)

59. The following characteristics are commonly seen in adolescents and relate to their developmental task according to Erikson. Which of the following statements does *not* relate?

A. use of peer group for support and identity
B. interest in religion
C. short-lived heterosexual relationships
D. family values have more importance than peer values (9:262,263)

60. A five-year-old boy puts up five fingers to indicate his age. This indicates the use of
A. preoperational behavior
B. concrete operations
C. sensorimotor operations
D. formal operations (3:238)

61. Certain behaviors develop and continue to be used because
A. they are useful in warding off anxiety
B. of normal maturational processes
C. they call out tenderness responses from adults
D. children cannot differentiate fantasy from consensually validated things (13:534)

62. Dramatizations enable children to learn about authority figures by acting like them, thus creating roles for themselves that
A. expose them to ridicule by others
B. avoid experiences with anxiety
C. call out tenderness responses
D. B and C (13:536)

63. Piaget postulated that in animistic ideation, the child tends to
A. connect sleep and death
B. regard everything as being controlled by men
C. regard objects as living and endowed with will
D. view death as irreversible (3:240,241)

64. In the second stage of animism, the child believes that
A. consciousness is restricted to animals
B. all things that move have consciousness
C. everything that moves is alive
D. things moving of their own accord have consciousness (3:232,233,234)

65. A four-year-old child who predominantly regards things as the product of human inventions reflects a developmental barrier that Piaget calls
A. egocentricity
B. rationalization
C. animism
D. artificialism (3:195,196,197)

66. What type of language is being demonstrated when a child is talking about himself, believing someone is listening, but has no desire to influence the hearer?
A. syntaxic
B. egocentric
C. parataxic
D. autistic (13:532)

67. The primary purpose of the aforenoted language is to
A. accompany and reinforce individual activity
B. communicate with peer group
C. adapt to the external environment
D. enjoy listening to oneself (3:176,177)

68. The primary task during adolescence is to develop a
A. degree of self-discipline
B. sense of right and wrong
C. lasting sense of well-being
D. firm sense of self (9:261)

69. Which of the following will be accomplished if a boy in late adolescence successfully completes his developmental tasks?
a. creation of a satisfactory relationship with girls
b. separation from parents and family
c. acceptance of his new body image
d. integration of his personality toward responsibility
e. decision concerning what vocation he will follow
A. a, b and c
B. b, d and e
C. c, d and e
D. All of the above (13:684)

70. The following characteristics are commonly seen in adolescents and relate to their developmental tasks according to Erikson.

Theoretical Perspectives

Which of the following statements does *not* relate?
A. use of peer group for support and identity
B. interest in religion
C. short-lived heterosexual relationships
D. use of symbolism (9:261)

71. Failure of the adolescent to establish a firm sense of self-identity will lead him to a state of
A. isolation
B. dependence
C. role confusion
D. despair (9:262)

72. Which of the following statements about a preschooler's growth and development is false?
A. all aspects of development are affected by the experiences in which the child finds himself
B. growth and development follows a definite, orderly pattern
C. each stage presents certain developmental tasks which the child may accomplish before going on to the next stage
D. his rate of development will be very similar to that of his 8-year-old brother (28:2,3)

73. Which of the following statements describes a child at 5 years of age?
a. enjoys parallel play
b. enjoys dramatic play
c. asks questions about birth and death
d. has a vocabulary of over 2000 words
e. can name basic colors
f. needs help in dressing himself
A. a, c, e and f
B. a, d, e and f
C. b, c, d and e
D. b, c, d and f (13:533,534)

74. Which of the following statements describe some developmental norms for a seven-year-old?
a. he has a decrease in rate of physical growth
b. he has increased small muscle coordination
c. he refuses to play with members of the opposite sex
d. he has all permanent teeth except his third molars
e. he prefers craftwork to outdoor activities
A. a, b and c
B. a, c and e
C. b, d and e
D. c, d and e (13:607,608,609)

75. The school-age child must develop a sense of industry and if he does not meet with success in his efforts he is very likely to develop a sense of
A. shame
B. guilt
C. inferiority
D. despair (9:260)

76. The development of basic trust in an infant depends primarily upon the quality of
A. birth process
B. mother-child relationship
C. health care delivery system
D. family relationships (13:280)

77. According to Erickson, the most serious danger for the adolescent is the failure to establish a sense of
A. identity and self-worth
B. initiative
C. industry
D. intimacy (3:371)

78. Which of the following is *not* characteristic of growth and development during the school years?
A. general growth is slow
B. child shows progressively slower growth in height, but rapid gain in weight
C. muscular coordination improves steadily
D. child shows progressively faster growth in height, but slower gain in weight (13:605)

79. The sixth year of development is best described as a (an)
A. assimilative age
B. year of transition

C. ambivalent period
D. quieting-down stage (13:606)

80. By the time the child reaches his sixth birthday, basically, he should have learned to trust others and should have developed a sense of
   A. identity
   B. intimacy
   C. industry
   D. autonomy (13:601)

81. According to Piaget, the developmental period characteristic of children aged 2 to 7 years is
   A. sensorimotor
   B. preoperational
   C. concrete
   D. formal (3:191)

82. Which of the following behaviors is indicative that the child is in the stage of concrete operations?
   A. distinguishes distance between two objects
   B. understands basic principles of casual thinking
   C. looks for object that "goes out of sight"
   D. uses simple tools to obtain objects (3:193)

83. The first step in cognitive representation according to Piaget is the
   A. symbolic schema
   B. verbal schema
   C. mental image
   D. perceptual image (3:230,231)

84. Jenny said "cry, cry" to her cat and she imitated the sound of crying. For Piaget, this behavior illustrates a child's
   A. identification of her body with that of other animals
   B. identification of one object with another
   C. projection of imitative schema onto new objects
   D. projection of symbolic schema onto new objects (3:233)

85. Psychoanalytic theory distinguishes between defenses and controls. The basic difference is that controls
   A. distort consciousness
   B. inhibit expression of and modify drive
   C. prevent expression of drive
   D. bring about altered motivations (3:355)

86. Freud postulated which one of the following as the cornerstone of all defenses?
   A. repression
   B. suppression
   C. intellectualization
   D. isolation (3:335,336)

87. A common accompaniment of repression is
   A. reaction-formation
   B. projection
   C. denial
   D. displacement (3:336)

88. Which of the following mechanisms is a protection against the acting-out of undesirable drives?
   A. projection
   B. displacement
   C. reaction-formation
   D. isolation (3:337,338)

89. According to the psychoanalytic theory, the ego functions in the following ways, *except*
   A. controls drives by delaying, inhibiting, and restraining them within context of realistic demands
   B. maximizes eventual gratification that comes from drive discharge
   C. reconciles incompatible impulses
   D. imposes system of norms and standards (3:319,320)

90. Which of the following statements does not accurately reflect the influence of sex upon growth and development?
   A. male infant is both longer and heavier than female infant
   B. girls mature earlier and so reach period of accelerated growth earlier than boys
   C. permanent teeth erupt earlier in boys than girls

D. bone development is more advanced in girls than in boys (13:27)

91. Probably the best gross index of nutrition and growth is
    A. weight
    B. height
    C. head circumference
    D. thoracic diameter (13:30)

92. Which one statement below does not reflect accurately the use of intelligence tests?
    A. intelligence tests during infancy and early childhood are useful only for showing general level of intelligence
    B. intelligence tests administered to infants and preschoolers are fair predictors of child's later intellectual attainment
    C. mental maturity is usually reached between ages 16 and 21 years
    D. there is higher degree of consistency in intelligence test results from age 5 onward than for tests given during preschool years (13:33)

93. The development of muscular control proceeds
    A. from head to cauda
    B. from head to periphery
    C. from center of body to periphery
    D. A and C (13:32)

94. Children with an I.Q. of 140 are considered to be
    A. average
    B. above-average
    C. gifted
    D. borderline (13:33)

95. Which one task below needs to be developed during the beginning years of adolescence? A sense of
    A. identity
    B. industry
    C. initiative
    D. intimacy (13:35)

96. Which group below is most likely to be the "significant others" of the school-age child?
    A. parental persons
    B. basic family
    C. peer group
    D. school (13:35)

97. Which of the following behaviors among adolescents is *not* suggestive that a sense of intimacy and solidarity has been established?
    A. boys losing interest in scouting
    B. girls losing interest in cliques of their own sex
    C. keeping relations with others on formal basis
    D. relating with own resources (13:35,36)

98. Training a child in the culture of the group reflects the process of
    A. in-breeding
    B. socialization
    C. discipline
    D. education (13:36)

99. Which developmental task below need *not* be a concern in the management of toddlers?
    A. sex information
    B. elimination control
    C. learning to talk
    D. learning social norms (13:419)

100. Between the ages of 6 and 12 years the child generally demonstrates the following behavior, *except*
    A. cooperating with others
    B. forming close ties of friendship
    C. conforming to social norms
    D. alternating conformity and rebellion against adult authority (13:601)

C. Developmental Correlates

Directions: For each of the following multiple choice questions, select the ONE most appropriate answer.

101. According to Gesell, assessment of the child can be divided into four fields of behavior. Which of the following is *not* one of these fields of behavior?
    A. language
    B. motor
    C. psychosexual
    D. personal-social (28:15)

102. Which is a true statement regarding the Denver Developmental Test?
    A. it can be used to test infants, preschool and school age children
    B. it indicates intelligence quotas
    C. it tests gross motor behavior
    D. it tests psychological behavior (13:24)

103. A 6-month-old infant would be expected to roll
    A. from supine to prone, sit without support, begin finger feeding
    B. from prone to supine, stand without support, relate willingly to strangers
    C. over completely, stand with support, spoon feed herself
    D. over completely, sit without support, reach for toy out of reach (13:291)

104. Which of the following characteristics would best describe a male at approximately 34 weeks gestation who weighs 2400 grams?
    A. flaccid muscle tone, weak grasp reflex, regular respirations, labile temperature
    B. tight muscle tone, weak grasp reflex, irregular respirations, labile temperature
    C. flaccid muscle tone, weak grasp reflex, irregular respirations, labile temperature
    D. tight muscle tone, weak grasp reflex, regular respirations, labile temperature (13:158,159)

105. Which of the following is true about a twelve-year-old boy?
    A. he has just gone through a period of rapid growth
    B. he will be expected to have a period of rapid growth in another 3 years
    C. he is gaining weight rapidly but growing very little
    D. he is expected to show little change in height or weight (13:680)

106. A girl, at 12 years of age, would show
    a. an increase in the diameter of the pelvis
    b. growth of pubic hair
    c. growth of axillary hair
    d. breast enlargement
    A. a, b and c
    B. a, b and d
    C. a, c and d
    D. b, c and d (13:689)

107. Which of the following would be typical behavior for a three month old?
    A. smiles in response to his mother's face, holds head erect
    B. rolls over completely, follows bright objects past the midline
    C. reaches for and transfers grasp of bright colored objects, recognizes his mother
    D. holds back straight when pulled to a sitting position, transfers objects from hand to hand (13:289)

108. A normal 36-week-old infant is now able to maintain a sitting position. He achieved head control at 24 weeks. According to Gesell's developmental theory, this developmental phenomena indicates
    A. increased complexity
    B. reciprocity
    C. rhythms and cycles
    D. synchrony (28:14,15,16,17)

109. Which are normal for a six-month-old child?
    a. closure posterior fontanels but not the anterior fontanels
    b. tonic neck reflex when lying down
    c. stares at hands when lying down
    d. large adenoids and tonsils
    e. palpable liver, 1–2 cm. below right costal margin
    f. unable to sit by himself
    A. a, b, d and e
    B. a, d and e
    C. b, d and f
    D. a, b, e and f (13:291,299)

110. A four-year-old child could be expected to
    a. button clothes and tie her shoes
    b. tell time and count to ten
    c. use a spoon and fork when eating
    d. pretend in her play and put away her toys
    A. a and b
    B. a and d
    C. b and c
    D. c and d (13:532)

111. Which of the following indicates the sequence of the development of language?
    A. jargon, vowel sounds, words
    B. words, jargon, sentence formation
    C. jargon, words, sentence formation
    D. vowel sounds, jargon, sentence formation (28:16,17)

112. All of the following are danger signals that should make a nurse think of disturbed interpersonal relations in an older child *except*
    A. failure to discriminate adequately between familiar and unfamiliar people
    B. difficulties in engaging in playful interchange with others at level expected of his age
    C. constriction of range and repertoire of positive and negative feelings
    D. none of above (10:129)

113. The capacity to play is frequently delayed if the child is suffering from the following conditions, *except*
    A. maternal deprivation
    B. consensual validation
    C. mental subnormality
    D. infantile psychosis (10:129)

115. In the second year, the dominant pleasure region is the
    A. anus
    B. mouth
    C. genitalia
    D. breasts (9:86-88)

116. Which of the following behaviors may *not* be expected in a four-month-old infant?
    A. smiles and wiggles body upon seeing milk bottle
    B. grasps objects and explores with mouth-hand-eyes coordination
    C. fixes gaze on mobile objects
    D. bites nipples (10:337)

117. Which of the following are basically anxiety-producing situations for a young child?
    A. fear of being abandoned by significant other
    B. fear of losing significant other's love
    C. fear of being punished
    D. A and B (10:339)

118. According to Robertson, a mother's adjustment to her new baby and his care should have reached a point by eight weeks of age at which time the mother shows the following behavior, *except*
    A. feels quite comfortable and competent about her mothering behavior
    B. able to "read" his feelings such as hunger and need for bodily contact reasonably well and response to them
    C. more anxious than usual during this period
    D. expresses pleasure in having her baby and in mothering him (10:340)

119. Which of the manifestations below is *not* considered normal for a one-month-old infant?
    A. gives heed to sounds
    B. turns head laterally when prone
    C. expresses differential cries for discomfort, pain and hunger
    D. stays put when prone on flat surfaces (28:15)

120. Which of the following behaviors can *not* be expected of a healthy baby at two years of age?
    A. builds tower of six to seven cubes
    B. tells experiences
    C. goes upstairs and downstairs alone
    D. refers to self by name (28:16)

121. Which of the following is generally *not* accomplished by three-year-old children?
    A. rides tricycle
    B. unbuttons buttons
    C. copies a square
    D. copies a circle (28:17)

122. Personal-social behavior in a normal nine-month-old baby is commonly demonstrated in
    A. waving bye-bye
    B. banging spoon on plate
    C. using both hands playfully
    D. turning pages of book (28:15)

123. A characteristic expression of a child's adaptive ability at six months of age is
    A. definitely looking for dropped spoon

B. giving definite attention to scribbling
 C. building tower of two blocks
 D. reaching for objects in sight   (28:15)

124. Which of the following is below Gesell's normative behavior for a one-year-old child?
 A. says two "words"
 B. repeats performance laughed at
 C. reacts to mirror image by manipulation
 D. holds crayon adaptively to make stroke   (28:15,16)

Directions: Match the following numbered items with the most appropriate lettered items, in relation to the behavioral expectations of a five-year-old boy.

125. Understands taking turns   (28:17)
126. Counts backward from 20 to 1   (28:17)
127. Begins to name colors   (28:17)
128. Skips using feet alternately   (28:17)
129. Names day of the week   (28:17)
130. Dresses and undresses self   (28:17)
131. Differentiates between right and left   (28:17)

 A. Expected
 B. Delayed
 C. Advanced
 D. Markedly advanced

Directions: Match the following numbered items with the most appropriate lettered items in relation to the growth and development of an eighteen-month-old girl.

132. Aligns cubes, imitating train   (28:16)
133. Says ten words, including name   (28:16)
134. Washes and dries face   (28:17)
135. Stands alone briefly   (28:16)
136. Takes feet to mouth persistently   (28:15)
137. Carries or hugs a special toy   (28:16)
138. Kicks large ball   (28:16)
139. Begins expressive jargon   (28:16)
140. Pulls toys on string   (28:16)
141. Carries out two directions   (28:16)

 A. The activity falls within the average for the age of this child
 B. The activity occurred earlier than in the average child
 C. The activity occurred later than in the average child
 D. The activity reflects possible severe mental retardation

Directions: For each of the following multiple choice questions, select the ONE most appropriate answer.

142. Which of the following is *not* true about weight?
 A. the usual range of birth weight is from 5–11 lbs.
 B. there is a physiological weight loss during the first 3 or 4 days of life which may be as much as 10% of birth weight
 C. at 1 year of age, birth weight is tripled
 D. at 10 years of age, weight is 10 times birth weight   (28:5)

143. The growth of the head is related to the growth of the
 A. nervous system
 B. brain
 C. spinal cord
 D. B and C   (28:5)

144. The lacrimal glands generally start secreting tears
 A. by the end of the first two months of life
 B. about the fourth month of life
 C. by the sixth week of life
 D. none of above   (28:6)

145. At birth the chest circumference is
 A. equal to head circumference
 B. about the same as that of abdominal circumference
 C. about one-half inch smaller than head
 D. B and C   (28:8)

146. Deciduous teeth are 20 in number. How many permanent teeth are there?
 A. 28
 B. 30
 C. 32
 D. 34   (28:8)

147. The glomerular filtration rate is low in the newborn. The adult rate is attained at what age?
 A. 4 years
 B. at about 2 years

C. at 6 years
D. at 10 years (28:11)

148. The low concentrating capacity of the kidney in infancy is probably due to the following factors, *except*
    A. low rate of urea and electrolyte excretion
    B. high rate of urea and electrolyte excretion
    C. shortness of loop of Henle
    D. none of above (28:11)

149. Height and weight increase steadily during the preschool years. The average gain per year in length is 3 inches and in weight
    A. 6 pounds
    B. 8 pounds
    C. 10 pounds
    D. none of above (10:389)

150. The increased capacity for locomotion and its integration with new mental and fine motor functions greatly increase the child's capacity
    A. to experience anxiety
    B. to adapt to new situations
    C. for exploration
    D. for initiative (10:389)

151. Which of the following standard developmental tests is particularly useful after six years of age?
    A. Gesell Developmental Schedules
    B. Stanford-Binet Scale
    C. Denver Developmental Screening Test
    D. none of above (10:389)

152. Which of the resources below are essentially adaptive devices for buffering the impact of stress upon a preschool child?
    A. ability to accept limits
    B. interest and warmth in social relations
    C. capacity to regress when needed
    D. all of above (10:391)

153. Which of the following statements is true about osseous development?
    A. females show earlier maturation
    B. rheumatoid arthritis may delay appearance of center
    C. precocious puberty causes a delay
    D. Caucasians have earlier maturation than Negroes (28:11,12)

Directions: Match the following numbered items with the most appropriate lettered items.

154. Pats mirror image (28:15)
155. Follows moving objects to midline (28:15)
156. Sits alone with good coordination (28:15)
157. Laughs aloud (28:15)
158. Symmetrical postures predominate (28:15)
159. Responds to "pat-a-cake" or "peek-a-boo" (28:15)
160. Beginning vocalization such as gurgling or grunting (28:15)
161. One-hand approach and grasp of toy (28:15)

    A. 4 weeks
    B. 16 weeks
    C. 28 weeks
    D. 40 weeks

Directions: For each of the following multiple choice questions, select the ONE most appropriate answer.

162. The normal bleeding time is
    A. 2–6 min.
    B. 1–3 min.
    C. 4–6 min.
    D. 5–8 min. (28:13)

163. The icterus index should be
    A. 5–10 units
    B. 6–8 units
    C. 6–12 units
    D. 3–5 units (28:13)

164. Which of the following values reflects a normal fasting blood sugar level?
    A. 5–7 mg/100 ml
    B. 5–40 units
    C. 60–120 mg/100 ml
    D. 60–120 units (28:13)

165. The potential for growth is greatest in which developmental period?
    A. conception
    B. infancy
    C. puberty
    D. adolescence (28:26)

166. Which of the following secondary sexual characteristics usually develops first in males?
    A. pubic hair
    B. deepening of voice
    C. increase in size of genitalia
    D. axillary hair (28:26)

167. The period of most rapid linear growth is
    A. 2 years of age to school age
    B. pubescence to 16 years of age
    C. birth to 2 years of age
    D. adolescence to maturity (28:26)

168. Which of the changes below occurs first in females?
    A. broadening of hips
    B. breast budding
    C. pubic hair
    D. axillary hair (28:26)

169. The hormones responsible for the appearance of secondary sex characteristics in males are
    A. gonadotropins
    B. androgens
    C. testosterones
    D. estrogens (28:26)

170. Which hormones stimulate the growth and development of ovaries and testes?
    A. gonadotropins
    B. androgens
    C. testosterones
    D. estrogens (28:26)

171. A child can repeat months in order, does simple division and multiplication, reads on own initiative and writes occasional short letters. The child is at least
    A. 7 years old
    B. 8 years old
    C. 9 years old
    D. 10 years old (28:17)

Directions: Match the following numbered items with the most appropriate lettered items.

172. Large-sized head for body size and age (1:40)
173. Facial grimace elicited when zygomatic bone is tapped (1:32)
174. Suture dividing right from left parietal bone (1:34)
175. First cervical vertebra supporting cranium (1:35)
176. Asymmetry of neck muscles causing head to be tilted to one side (1:42)
177. Lack of hair in spots (1:41)
178. Soft, fluctuating mass of blood trapped beneath pericranium and confined to one bone (1:38)
179. Close-set eyes, with a small nasal bridge (1:43)
180. Unossified membranous intervals of infant skull (1:34)
181. Resonant, cracked-pot sound, heard upon percussing child's skull with increased intracranial pressure (1:43)

    A. Sagittal suture
    B. Alopecia
    C. Hypotelorism
    D. Macrocephaly
    E. Cephalhematoma
    F. Fontanels
    G. Chvostek's sign
    H. Atlas
    I. Torticollis
    J. Macewen's sign
    K. Oxycephaly
    L. Coronal suture

Directions: For each of the following multiple choice questions, select the ONE most appropriate answer.

182. What suture separates the parietal bones from the occipital bone?
    A. lambdoidal suture
    B. sagittal suture
    C. coronal suture
    D. frontal suture (1:34)

183. The suture that goes from ear to ear across the top of the skull is the
 A. lambdoidal suture
 B. sagittal suture
 C. coronal suture
 D. frontal suture (1:34)

184. The spaces between the skull bones are called
 A. fontanels
 B. sutures
 C. junctions
 D. cavities (1:34)

185. The skull is divided into two sections, the cranium and the
 A. fontanels
 B. sutures
 C. epicranium
 D. facial skeleton (1:33)

186. Which of the following is not a cranial bone?
 A. frontal bone
 B. temporal bone
 C. occipital bone
 D. sphenoid bone (1:33,34)

187. The skin covering the subcutaneous fascia and muscle on the skull is
 A. thicker than on any other part of the body
 B. thinner than on any other part of the body
 C. as thick as any other part of the body
 D. more vascular than any other part of the body (1:36)

188. The most important nerves supplying the face and head are the
 A. sympathetic nerves
 B. parasympathetic nerves
 C. cranial nerves
 D. trigeminal nerves (1:37)

189. Which of the following statements is *not* about the thyroid gland?
 A. it is an extremely vascular endocrine gland
 B. it has no ducts and secretes hormones directly into the bloodstream
 C. it secretes thyroxin which is essential for normal body growth
 D. it is larger in males than in females (1:37)

190. Most infants are born with 6 fontanels but the most prominent are the
 A. anterior and posterior
 B. mastoid and sphenoid
 C. anterior and mastoid
 D. posterior and sphenoid (1:34)

191. The only movable facial bone is the
 A. zygomatic
 B. maxilla
 C. mandible
 D. temporal (1:34)

192. The vertebra that is used for identification when palpating the spinal column is the
 A. sixth
 B. seventh
 C. eighth
 D. ninth (1:35)

193. Blood circulation for the head and neck is supplied through the
 A. jugular veins
 B. carotid veins
 C. jugular arteries
 D. carotid arteries (1:37)

194. Frontal bulges are known as *bossing* in infants and this may be the first indication of
 A. scurvy and leprosy
 B. syphilis and rickets
 C. Kwashiorkor and Tay-Sach's disease
 D. none of the above (1:38)

195. A small rounded depression in the frontal and parietal bones in newborns is a
 A. normal result of the birth process
 B. sign of Hurler's syndrome
 C. sign of skull fracture
 D. sign of rickets (1:38)

Chapter II: Answers and Explanations

1. **B.**—The greatest rates of growth take place during fetal life, infancy and adolescence.
2. **C.**—The only child being constantly with adults, particularly with his parents, can very well be mentally stimulated by their companionship.
3. **D.**—While the child has his own potentiality for growth, his individual pattern of growth and development is determined by the interplay of heredity and environmental factors.
4. **A.**—The first slow period of growth occurs from 2 years of age to pubescence.
5. **C.**—These seasonal variations in height and weight reflect the impact of season as a factor influencing growth.
6. **B.**—Maturation is often used interchangeably with development; however, maturation is generally referred to as development of traits carried through the genes.
7. **C.**—Euthenics aims at establishing a wholesome environment for all age groups.
8. **A.**—Development implies specialization of functions.
9. **B.**—Stereophotogrammetry is the technique employed.
10. **A.**—Physioprinting is the technique employed for guiding in tooth-straightening and denture filling.
11. **D.**—Developmental examinations bear a *low* predictability of later mental functioning and as such should not be considered as a test of intelligence.
12. **B.**—If repeated measurements are taken, it is possible to determine whether the percentile position at any one time represents the normal pattern for that individual or suggests some pathologic condition.
13. **C.**—*After* puberty, the trunk grows slightly faster than the extremities.
14. **B.**—The principle of reciprocy postulates the inseparability of man and environment.
15. **A.**—The principle of helicy subsumes within it the principles of reciprocy and synchrony and emphasizes the unitary nature of the man-environment relationship.
16. **A.**—Rhythmicity characterizes both the human field and the environmental field and the pattern of the human field is a wave phenomenon encompassing man in his entirety.
17. **D.**—The capacity of man and his environment to engage in a continuous interaction process rests on the fact that both are demonstrably open systems.
18. **C.**—The principle of homeostasis is aimed at attaining a state of relative equilibrium of man's internal regulatory states in the midst of constant flux in the environment; as such it contradicts the principles of homeodynamics.
19. **B.**—The principle of helicy basically assumes that the life process is characterized by probabilistic goal-directedness.
20. **C.**—Early adolescence is found to bear the greatest potential for growth and this stage is important in estimating final height.
21. **D.**—Girls start adolescence at about 10 years of age, while boys start at about 12 years.
22. **A.**—If a lie is told, the child will lose his sense of trust in the individual and his trust in all others may be weakened.
23. **C.**—A child sees the reality of the birth of a sibling and resolves the situation by

healthfully seeking pleasure with his peer group rather than clinging on to his mother.
24. **B.**—The child is internally motivated to do things which will give him a sense of worth.
25. **A.**—These children learn early that some are given opportunities and restrictions while others are not.
26. **C.**—The child is at an expansive age and wants to do everything.
27. **D.**—The desired behavior will occur consistently when subsequently reinforced at intermittent occasions.
28. **A.**—These children have unusually large vocabularies and a facility of expression.
29. **C.**—Intelligence testing in the preschool period, or earlier, is generally not appropriate.
30. **C.**—Parents and others involved should not permit a child to overschedule himself in various extracurricular activities or to feel excessively pushed at school or at home.
31. **D.**—Responding emotionally to family members may be attained as early as seven or eight months of age.
32. **A.**—Through conditioning, the infant learns to eliminate when placed on toilet and with maturation the child learns to express his needs and assumes a degree of responsibility for them.
33. **C.**—Children of this age are quite sensitive about sex and avoid self-exposure in front of the opposite sex.
34. **D.**—Development of short-term attachments with members of the opposite sex which tend to break up the intense friendship with members of the same sex may be a fairly reliable indicator of his future sexual orientation.
35. **A.**—Sporadic homosexual experience during this period may be viewed as age-specific, even age-appropriate.
36. **B.**—An individual is apt to have no strong role model if he belongs to a family that did not foster self-esteem. Young people can also be remarkably clannish in their exclusion of all those who are "outside" of their group.
37. **C.**—Adolescents not only help one another temporarily, through the formation of cliques and by stereotyping themselves and their enemies; they also test each other's capacity to pledge fidelity.
38. **A.**—The adolescent's ideas are dominated by the social and ethical codes in the group. Fads are important. He may not express his individuality beyond the limits imposed by the groups. Peers share each other's ideas, deepest secrets and troubles, thereby developing a strong sense of responsibility and loyalty to others.
39. **C.**—Children in this age group have a strong sense of duty. They want to engage in tasks in their social world which they can carry out successfully and they want their success to be recognized by the surrounding adults and by their peers.
40. **A.**—Perceiving consciousness as present only in animals reflects intuitive operations.
41. **C.**—The 3-year-old child talks in sentences about things. He does not appear to care whether others listen or not.
42. **A.**—In the preoperational stage, the child uses *intuition* instead of logic.
43. **D.**—All the enumerated behaviors serve as a basis for the preschooler's sense of initiative.
44. **A.**—Limit setting and encouragement are apt to give a child a sense of security which is essential to the development of self-esteem.
45. **D.**—All the aforenoted experiences are some of the rational operations reflective of the concrete phase of cognitive development.
46. **D.**—The adolescent may be expected to select and prepare for an occupation rather than get started in one.
47. **D.**—Three kinds of vocation face the young person: the vocation of citizenship, the vocation which will make a living for himself and his family, and the vocation of parenthood. Adolescents should be prepared for prospective problems involved in each.
48. **A.**—Developing basic trust is the crucial developmental task of infancy.
49. **C.**—By the time the child is 12 years old, he should have developed positive attitudes toward his own and other social, racial, economic and religious groups aside from having learned the concepts necessary for daily living.

50. **D.**—Girls may spend hours making themselves more attractive and learn to cook, clean and sew. Boys are usually interested in competing and excelling in sports.
51. **B.**—The attitudes and feelings which children acquire greatly influence their relations with marital partners and with their own children later.
52. **C.**—Limits to the child's behavior must be relatively set and consistently maintained to provide a basis for predicting the reactions of other people to what he does and says.
53. **A.**—This is a very important developmental task as this marks the child's newly evolved independence reflecting a beginning mastery of motor apparatus, including both movement and language, and an emerging ability to assess reality.
54. **B.**—Reality testing can be described as one of the ego functions which is based on the child's capacity, more or less, to tell whether something is "self" or "non-self".
55. **B.**—The manifest dream content may or may not be remembered upon awakening. Freud believed that there are universal symbols used in dream work and one could gain knowledge of the person's unconscious by decoding his manifest dreams.
56. **C.**—Freud postulated that daydreams are carried out in thought and don't take the form of a hallucinatory experience.
57. **C.**—The anal stage provides the child an opportunity to learn much about his body and experience some of his capacities, limitations and power. It is considered more favorable for future development if he is allowed to express his hostility toward the parent directly.
58. **D.**—Freud believed that castration fears change a boy's relationship to his father and bring out nurtual ambivalence. Under pressure of guilt feelings, a boy will attempt to intensify his dependence on his father and try to please him.
59. **D.**—Adolescents stereotype themselves, their ideals, and many other things and as such would see family values as being less important than peer values.
60. **A.**—Affect, action, and thought are closely interrelated during the preoperational phase. When the child struggles with the notion that a word is a label for a class of objects or actions, he meets for the first time the necessity for understanding a genuine concept.
61. **A.**—In this situation, it is significant to explore the underlying factors for such behavior.
62. **B.**—This is an expression of the child's "as if" performance which is an essential mechanism for future development.
63. **C.**—Animism is a concept which further supports Piaget's contention that the child's world is dominated by egocentrism.
64. **B.**—The child then believes that everything that moves is alive and finally comes to believe that consciousness is restricted to animals.
65. **D.**—During this period the child projects onto all things the relationship which he feels exists between himself and his parents.
66. **B.**—Egocentric speech is one of Piaget's two broad categories of language development which he hypothesized as predominantly operating up to age 7.
67. **A.**—Its adaptive value to the child is through assimilation.
68. **D.**—A firm sense of self is the accrued confidence that the inner sameness and continuity prepared in the past are matched by the sameness and continuity of one's meanings for others.
69. **D.**—All the aforenoted developmental tasks must be accomplished for the adolescent to grow into wholesome adult life.
70. **D.**—Use of symbolism is characteristic of the childhood years.
71. **C.**—The outcome of the adolescent's struggle to establish his sense of identity is dependent largely on his childhood experiences. Although the sense of identity is difficult to achieve, he must gain it in order to be saved from emotional turmoil.
72. **D.**—A preschooler's rate of growth and development would be different from that of an eight-year-old brother, for two individuals are not alike.
73. **C.**—A five-year-old child can be expected to dress and undress himself without assistance as well as play competitive exercise games.

Theoretical Perspectives

74. **A.**—A seven-year-old child truly prefers outdoor activities to craftwork.
75. **C.**—If the child fails in the use of his tools and skills or if his status among his peers is threatened, he may be discouraged from identifying with them or with the tool world.
76. **B.**—Inasmuch as the mother is generally the constant adult in the infant's life, the relationship between them makes a very strong impact upon the infant's life processes.
77. **A.**—The adolescent is faced with a choice of a whole way of life in terms of his job, political activities, his ethics, etc.
78. **D.**—A child tends to lose the thin, wiry appearance of the earlier years; posture should be good.
79. **B.**—The sixth year is a year of transition, of physical and psychologic changes, which determine whether the child is ready to enter school or not.
80. **D.**—He should also have developed a sense of initiative, but his activities should be partly controlled by his conscience.
81. **B.**—This is the period during which the child's internal cognitive picture of the external world, with its many laws and relationships, is gradually growing.
82. **A.**—The child, during the stage of concrete operations, acquires a rudimentary concept of time, space, number and logic.
83. **C.**—For Piaget, a mental image is not an image unless the child distinguishes it from a perception. He must differentiate the image from what it pictures.
84. **D.**—Such behavior reflects the earliest stage in the development of symbolic schemas as they appear in the play of the preschool child.
85. **B.**—Controls otherwise tame the drive without bringing about any alteration of its basic nature.
86. **A.**—Accordingly, all other defenses are associated with some degree of repression.
87. **D.**—The significant feature about the displacement mechanism is that the behavior resorted to does not arouse anxiety that the primary behavior would.
88. **C.**—Reaction-formation consists of the establishment of a drive derived out of the countercathexis which prevents the appearance of the repressed material. Thus, hostility is overtly replaced by excessive kindness.
89. **D.**—The superego imposes a system of norms and standards and roles quite independently of individual happiness.
90. **C.**—Girls demonstrate advance in osseous development as may be reflected in earlier eruption of the permanent teeth.
91. **A.**—Weight is influenced by all the increments in size. Excess weight in relation to the height and pelvic diameter is as abnormal as being underweight.
92. **B.**—Intelligence tests administered to infants and preschoolers are of the performance type and as such show only the general level of intelligence. They do not accurately predict the child's later intellectual attainment.
93. **D.**—Muscular control does not develop evenly throughout the body. It follows the principle of cephalo-caudal direction and proceeds from the center of the body to the periphery.
94. **C.**—An I.Q. between 90 and 109 is usually considered average and anything less than average represents retardation of varying degrees.
95. **A.**—This period is characterized by the adolescent's attitude toward life as "What will this mean to me?"
96. **D.**—Society reaches the child directly through the school system and educates him intellectually and in the fundamental skills of living in a modern society.
97. **C.**—This type of relationship with others lacks warmth, and if persistently demonstrated, the adolescent is eventually led to a psychological isolation.
98. **B.**—Love and consistency in training are necessary to socialize the child.
99. **A.**—Sex information is most appropriate during the preschool years as this is the period when the child is initially aware of the differentiation of sexes and demonstrates substantial interest in exploring his own body.
100. **B.**—The school years mark the development of a child's strong desire to engage in reality-oriented tasks.

101. **C.**—The other field of behavior included in child assessment, according to Gesell, is the adaptive field.
102. **C.**—The use of the Denver Developmental Screening Test is limited only to infants and preschool children. Aside from testing gross motor behavior, it evaluates motor-adaptive areas and language and personal-social areas.
103. **A.**—The 6-month-old infant pulls himself up to a sitting position and sits momentarily without support if placed in a favorable leaning position.
104. **C.**—The premature infant's problems reflect the physiologic handicaps of immaturity such as inability to control body temperature, difficult respiration and inability to handle infections.
105. **B.**—Girls begin their preadolescent growth spurt by about ten years and boys by about twelve years.
106. **D.**—Girls *only* show an increase in the *transverse* diameter of the pelvis.
107. **A.**—At 3 months of age, in the area of socialization, the child also laughs aloud and shows pleasure in making sounds.
108. **A.**—Increasing complexity in growth is associated with increasing functional differentiation of body organs hence, specialization of functions.
109. **B.**—The 6-month-old child should be a cause of concern if he still is assuming the tonic neck reflex or stares at hands when lying down or is unable to sit by himself.
110. **D.**—The 4-year-old child is generally too young to button clothes and tie shoes or tell time.
111. **C.**—Language development proceeds from vocalization, jargon, words, and then on to sentence formation.
112. **D.**—The three aforenoted behaviors are truly indicative of disturbed interpersonal relations in an older child.
113. **B.**—Consensual validation is an operational level of language development reflective of the child's ability to interpret events within the social context, thus facilitating his ability to play with others.
114. **C.**—Play enables a child to deal with anxiety-laden situations on a therapeutic level.
115. **A.**—The child is in the anal stage of psychosexual development and uses the anus also for release of aggression.
116. **D.**—Biting nipples usually takes place in the second six months of life, as the infant expresses aggressive feelings toward feeding regimentation.
117. **D.**—Fear of being abandoned and losing the love of "significant other" have been recognized as the two fundamental danger situations that produce anxiety. The ego of the child is strongly influenced by his inner fantasy world rather than the external reality.
118. **A.**—While the mother, by eight weeks postpartum, finds pleasure in having her baby and in mothering him, she has not reached the point where she can feel quite comfortable and competent in mothering and caretaking.
119. **D.**—The one-month-old infant ordinarily makes crawling movements when prone on flat surface.
120. **B.**—That behavior is too advanced for a two-year-old child.
121. **C.**—Copying a square is too advanced for a three-year-old child; this can be expected of a five-year-old child.
122. **A.**—The other three forms of personal-social behavior generally take place in other periods; B and C anywhere from around five to six months and D around eighteen months.
123. **D.**—That is a behavior usually attained by seven months of age.
124. **D.**—The first three choices represent fairly advanced behavior.
125. **A.**—Such behavior is generally attained by three years of age.
126. **D.**—That is generally accomplished by eight years of age.
127. **B.**—A four-year-old child can very well be expected to demonstrate such behavior.
128. **A.**—That behavior, indeed, can be expected of a five year old.
129. **D.**—Naming days of the week is too advanced for this age level. This is ordinarily accomplished by seven years of age.
130. **A.**—That is a personal-social behavior that can be expected of five year olds.

131. **C.**—That behavior is usually accomplished by six years of age.
132. **B.**—This activity occurs generally by two years of age.
133. **A.**—The child is functioning optimally.
134. **B.**—This activity is a markedly advanced behavior, as it is usually attained by four year olds.
135. **C.**—By 1½ years of age, the child should be able to walk and seldom fall.
136. **D.**—This behavior should be a cause of concern. This may very well be engaged by seven-month-old babies.
137. **A.**—That is a healthy behavior for eighteen-month-old children.
138. **B.**—The ability to kick a large ball is generally attained by two years of age.
139. **C.**—That is a delayed behavior, for it is ordinarily attained by one year olds.
140. **A.**—The activity is a very enjoyable one for eighteen-month-old infants.
141. **A.**—Usually eighteen month olds can follow such directions as "give to mother" and "put on table."
142. **A.**—The usual range of birth weight is 6 to 9½ lbs.; the average being 7½ lbs.
143. **B.**—The importance of an accurate examination of the head in infants cannot be overemphasized; any deviation from the expected growth may indicate neuromotor disorder or abnormality such as microcephaly.
144. **A.**—Tears may not be produced before the third month of life.
145. **D.**—At 1 year of age, the chest circumference is equal to or exceeds the head circumference slightly.
146. **C.**—There are 32 permanent teeth which may be completed at 22 years of age.
147. **B.**—The glomerular rate change corresponds to the morphologic maturation of the kidney.
148. **B.**—Low rate of urea and electrolyte elimination as well as the shortness of the loop of Henle are probably factors explaining the low concentrating capacity of the kidney in infancy.
149. **D.**—The average yearly weight gain in the preschool age is 5 pounds.
150. **C.**—The child's increasing capacity for exploration can account for the rapid learning characterizing the preschool age group.
151. **D.**—None of the choices are right. The Stanford-Binet is a psychological test; the Gesell Developmental Schedules and the Denver Developmental Screening tests are good only in infancy and preschool years.
152. **D.**—Excessive use of such mechanisms may constitute maladaptive solutions to realistic integrative tasks.
153. **A.**—The given phenomena connote that sex is an influential factor in bone maturation.
154. **C.**—This is an aspect of personal-social behavior attained at about 28 weeks of age.
155. **A.**—This behavior can be expected of a 4-week-old infant.
156. **D.**—A healthy 40-week-old infant should be able to demonstrate this behavior.
157. **B.**—A 16-week-old infant ordinarily laughs aloud when actively played with by his mother or other familiar person.
158. **B.**—At 16 weeks of age the tonic neck reflex position is only seldom assumed by a healthy infant.
159. **D.**—This is the average age level when a child responds to social play.
160. **A.**—Associated with these vocalizations is cooing, which is also hardly sustained.
161. **C.**—Such activity is one of the dimensions of adaptive behavior at 28 weeks of age.
162. **B.**—Prolongation in bleeding time can result in hemorrhage which may prove fatal.
163. **D.**—Once the level gets higher than 5 units, the skin and sclera appear jaundiced.
164. **C.**—A higher level would indicate hyperglycemia and a lower level, hypoglycemia.
165. **D.**—The adolescent period is thus a very significant period in estimating final height.
166. **C.**—Sexual characteristics usually develop in a particular order, although there are differences in age of onset.
167. **B.**—Growth is accelerated during the period of sexual development and decelerates at sexual maturity when sex hormones influence the closing of epiphyses.
168. **A.**—Broadening of the hips occurs first followed by budding of the breast and then by appearance of pubic hair.
169. **B.**—Androgens are basically responsible

for secondary sexual characteristics in males.
170. **A.**—Gonadotropins are the influencing hormones.
171. **C.**—The child's performance is predominantly reflective of an average 9-year-old child.
172. **D.**—A small-size head for body size and age is called microcephaly.
173. **G.**—Chvostek's sign is positive if that side of the face shows a grimace. It is present in children normally under 1 month of age and over 5 years.
174. **A.**—The coronal suture goes from ear to ear across the top of the skull.
175. **H.**—The atlas, together with the axis, form a pivot for rotation of the head.
176. **I.**—The neck should be symmetrical from all angles.
177. **B.**—Alopecia may be familial or due to ringworm; it may also be a sign of hair pulling, or may be an indication of emotional problems.
178. **E.**—Cephalohematoma, or bleeding below the periosteum of the skull bones, may indicate a skull fracture.
179. **C.**—In contrast, hypertelorism reflects wide-set eyes with a broad flat nasal bridge.
180. **F.**—Most infants are born with 6 fontanels, but the most prominent are the anterior and the posterior.
181. **J.**—In an infant with an open fontanel, this sound is normal, but once the fontanels are closed the sound is indicative of a pathologic condition.
182. **A.**—The lambdoidal suture runs at an obtuse angle to the sagittal suture posteriorly.
183. **C.**—This suture runs at a right angle to the sagittal suture anteriorly.
184. **B.**—Sutures are frequently palpable at birth.
185. **D.**—The facial bones number 14 and are immovable except for the mandible.
186. **D.**—The sphenoid bone is one of the facial bones.
187. **A.**—The scalp has five tightly packed layers including the pericranium.
188. **C.**—There are 12 pairs of cranial nerves.
189. **D.**—Sex is not a factor in influencing size of the thyroid gland.
190. **A.**—Some infants have an additional fontanel along the sagittal suture between the anterior and the posterior. This is present in some children wih Down's syndrome, but can also be present in normal infants.
191. **C.**—At birth, the mandible and maxilla are very small, giving the head a flat, squashed face.
192. **B.**—The seventh vertebra has a long spinous process.
193. **D.**—The internal carotid supplies the structures within the cranium, while the external carotid carries blood to the head, face and neck.
194. **B.**—Any prominent bulge or swelling should be observed and felt for size, location and density.
195. **A.**—Caput succedaneum, or edema of the scalp, which generally crosses suture lines is noted on some infants following the birth process. Symmetry of the head and face is usually regained by the end of the first week.

CHAPTER III

Health Maintenance and Promotion

INTRODUCTION

Health nursing is an important component of family-centered nursing practice. In pediatric nursing, it addresses itself to total health needs and the welfare of children within the context of the family-community system. Likewise, it defines the roles and activities of the nurse in health maintenance and promotion. The increasing sophistication of diagnostic procedures and preventive measures for the control of diseases and other handicapping conditions constitutes a springboard for numerous activities to promote positive health. Health promotion connotes not only preventing the occurrence of illnesses, thus sustaining health, but above all it aims at assisting children and their parents to attain the highest levels of well-being possible.

Health nursing utilizes an orderly approach to health care through assessment, intervention, and evaluation ultimately aimed at building a healthful and dynamic society. Today's nurse acts as a practitioner, a health consultant, educator, counselor, interpreter, and evaluator. These different roles should take cognizance of the interrelationships of the many factors influencing individual and family growth and development.

This chapter deals with basic considerations that a nurse should be aware of in order to be an effective health facilitator. Substantial attention is given to health assessments, as these are crucial to planning and implementing appropriate nursing actions. While the indivisibility of all aspects of health is truly recognized for purposes of clarity and organization, health assessments are presented in two broad categories: physical and psychosocial assessments. Selected aspects of physical assessments are excluded since they are integrated in other sections of the book. Other areas covered herein are: screening tests, immunization, nutrition, dental supervision, communication, health education and counseling.

A. Physical Assessment

Directions: For each of the following multiple choice questions, select the ONE most appropriate answer.

1. A newborn is admitted to the newborn nursery directly from the delivery room. Which of the following is *not* true in relation to the condition of his normal umbilicus?

    A. clear whitish appearance
    B. slight pulse present
    C. presence of three blood vessels
    D. moist   (13:130,138)

2. An apgar rating of 7 means that the baby
    A. is average in his initial adjustment
    B. needs special attention
    C. is seriously depressed
    D. is probably premature   (13:127)

3. Asymmetry of the buttock and resistance to abduction in a newborn lead you to suspect
   A. tibial torsion
   B. dislocated hip *(circled)*
   C. developmental lag
   D. A and B   (13:267)

4. Which of the following is a deviation from normal characteristics of a newborn?
   A. bluish sclera
   B. chest approximately same circumference as the head
   C. molding
   D. closed posterior fontanel *(circled)*   (1:40)

5. Due to passage of hormones from the mother, certain characteristics may be noted in the newborn. Which of the following is *not* one?
   A. pseudomenstruation
   B. genital hypertrophy in males *(circled)*
   C. genital hypertrophy in females
   D. breast engorgement in males   (13:120,121)

6. Two days after birth, white patches in the infant's mouth were noticed before his feeding. This indicates which of the following problems?
   A. Epstein's pearls
   B. pseudostrabismus *(circled)*
   C. thrush *(circled)*
   D. pterygoid ulcers   (1:107)

7. A child's birth weight is 7½ lbs. At one year he should weigh approximately
   A. 14 lbs.
   B. 18 lbs.
   C. 22 lbs. — *triple 7½ × 3 = 22*
   D. 26 lbs.   (28:5)

8. The average adult requires a quart of water per day. The infant needs at least one-third as much water. His need is proportionally greater because
   A. the infant's body metabolism is more rapid *(circled)*
   B. more of the infant's body fluids are intracellular
   C. the infant has less body surface area in proportion to the adult
   D. the infant's immature kidneys conserve excessive water   (13:335)

9. What percentage of an infant's total body weight is composed of water?
   A. 40–49%
   B. 50–59%   *53% – adult*
   C. 60–69%
   D. 70–80% *(circled)*   (13:335)

10. In appraising a healthy one-month-old infant, the nurse should expect him to
    a. have gross, generalized movements
    b. have regular, abdominal respirations
    c. turn his head from side to side when in a prone position
    d. follow a bright object past the midline
    A. a and b
    B. a and c
    C. b and d
    D. c and d *(circled)*   (13:286)

11. The basic methods of physical examination include the following except
    A. inspection
    B. percussion
    C. auscultation
    D. smelling *(circled)*   (1:6)

12. The method of determining the density of various parts of the body by the sounds emitted by these parts when struck directly with the examiner's fingers is called
    A. inspection
    B. smelling
    C. percussion *(circled)*
    D. auscultation   (1:7)

13. Different parts of the hands are used for examining different sensations. Which parts of the hands are most sensitive to temperature?
    A. finger tips
    B. back of fingers *(circled)*
    C. palms
    D. flat of fingers   (1:6)

Health Maintenance and Promotion

14. The most useful method of physical examination, although it is often difficult to learn, is
    A. inspection
    B. smelling
    C. percussion
    D. auscultation (1:6)

15. Physical examination can be done under many conditions, but it is *always* preferable to secure
    A. some privacy
    B. proper equipment
    C. sufficient time for nurse and child to become comfortable in setting
    D. all of the above (1:3)

16. If the child appears frightened even before you have started the physical examination, he should be
    A. encouraged to sit on his mother's lap
    B. allowed to play quietly with some toys while mother is interviewed
    C. allowed to cry while you conduct the procedure
    D. A and B (1:3)

17. Which of the following is the least helpful technique in examining preschoolers?
    A. remove clothing one piece at a time allowing child to do as much as possible
    B. undress child all at once, thus speeding up procedure
    C. enlist child's help in examination whenever possible
    D. begin with certain tests for neurologic functions (1:5)

18. When examining an infant, it is usually best to begin with the
    A. feet and work toward head
    B. head and work toward feet
    C. trunk and work toward feet, then to head
    D. trunk and work toward head, then to feet (1:4)

19. When there are several children in the family to be examined on the same day, which type of child should be examined first?
    A. least fearful
    B. oldest
    C. youngest
    D. most anxious (1:7)

20. Which of the techniques below is likely to be *most* anxiety-provoking when examining an older child?
    A. allow him to hold or squeeze a toy during examination
    B. allow him to hold stethoscope or listen to his own heart through it
    C. ask him questions, only after examination has been completed
    D. show him otoscope and show how light turns on and off (1:6)

Directions: Match the following numbered items with the most appropriate lettered items.

21. Anterior portion of maxilla bone separating nasal and oral cavities (1:96)
22. Fungal inspection caused by candida albicans (1:107)
23. Infection of tongue (1:108)
24. Tooth decay leading to destruction of tooth (1:106)
25. Foul breath (1:105)
26. Retention cysts found in gums of newborn (1:105,106,107)
27. Cracked, bleeding lips (1:104)
28. Cold sore (1:110)
29. Tongue whose attachment is more forward than usual (1:107)
30. Inability to swallow (1:107)

    A. Hard palate
    B. Cheilitis
    C. Epstein pearls
    D. Caries
    E. Glossitis
    F. Dysphagia
    G. Thrush
    H. Glossoptosis
    I. Halitosis
    J. Soft palate
    K. Koplick's spots
    L. Herpes simplex

Directions: For each of the following multiple choice questions, select the ONE most appropriate answer.

31. The primary blood supply to the mouth is the
    A. external carotid artery
    B. internal carotid artery
    C. coronary artery
    D. subclavian artery (1:96)

32. Innervation of the oral cavity is supplied by which of the following cranial nerves?
    A. fifth cranial nerve
    B. fourth cranial nerve
    C. seventh cranial nerve
    D. A and C (1:97)

33. In which of the following structures is the epiglottis contained?
    A. pharynx
    B. oropharynx
    C. larynx
    D. laryngopharynx (1:98)

34. Which is the largest of the salivary glands?
    A. submandibular
    B. sublingual
    C. parotid
    D. adenoid (1:98)

35. Salivation begins at what age?
    A. 2 months
    B. 3 months
    C. 4 months
    D. 10 weeks (1:99)

36. Which part of the tooth is the exposed portion?
    A. crown — enamel
    B. neck
    C. root
    D. A and B (1:100)

37. Every child gets how many deciduous teeth?
    A. 32
    B. 28
    C. 24
    D. 20 (1:100)

38. All deciduous teeth should be erupted by what age?
    A. 3 years
    B. 2½ years
    C. 2 years
    D. 1½ years (1:100)

39. Usually the lower incisors are shed around what age?
    A. 4 years
    B. 5 years
    C. 6 years
    D. 7 years (1:00)

40. A child with pale lips and gums may be suffering from
    A. congenital heart disease
    B. anemia
    C. acidosis
    D. carbon monoxide poisoning (1:104)

41. Which of the following *does not* produce halitosis?
    A. poor oral hygiene, mouth breathing
    B. systemic infection, sinusitis
    C. mouth breathing, foreign body stuck in nose
    D. none of the above (1:105)

42. Which of the following diseases gives off ammoniacal odor?
    A. diphtheria
    B. typhoid fever
    C. uremia
    D. diabetic acidosis (1:105)

43. Discoloration of teeth can be due to several factors. Mottled and pitted teeth come from
    A. excess iron ingestion
    B. excess fluoride in drinking water
    C. tetracycline treatment
    D. B and C (1:106)

44. The classic sign of scarlet fever is
    A. Epstein pearls
    B. white, strawberry tongue
    C. beefy, red swollen tongue
    D. Koplick's spots (1:108)

45. Deviation of the tongue to one side may indicate a neoplasm on one side of tongue or an impairment of which cranial nerve?
    A. eighth
    B. ninth
    C. tenth
    D. twelfth (1:108)

The Nose

46. Another name for bleeding from the nose is
    A. epistaxis
    B. hemoptysis
    C. chemosis
    D. sclerosis (1:94)

47. Which of the paranasal sinuses are the largest?
    A. ethmoid
    B. frontal
    C. maxillary
    D. sphenoid (1:94)

48. The nostrils are otherwise called
    A. meatus
    B. nares
    C. conchae
    D. antrum of Highmore (1:94)

49. Which of the following structures of the respiratory system is *not* accessible to physical examination by the nurse?
    A. nose
    B. nasal passages
    C. larynx
    D. paranasal sinuses (1:86)

50. Which of the following muscles is used to wrinkle the nose?
    A. nasalis
    B. depressor septi
    C. median septum
    D. procerus (1:87)

51. Which of the following paranasal sinuses is *not* present at birth?
    A. frontal
    B. maxillary
    C. ethmoid
    D. sphenoid (1:89)

52. Examination of the child's nose is best approached when he is in which of the following positions?
    A. lying on his back on the table
    B. sitting either on table or mother's lap
    C. Fowler's position on table
    D. standing (1:90)

53. Which of the following signs usually results from chronic rhinitis
    A. inflammation and erythema of nasal mucosa
    B. pale, boggy mucosa
    C. swollen, gray mucosa
    D. B and C (1:90)

54. Which of the following factors accounts for the largest percentage of nosebleeds?
    A. trauma to the nose
    B. high dry altitude
    C. hypertension, tuberculosis, kidney disease
    D. exposure to certain chemical fumes (1:93)

55. Which of the following measures is *not* advisable for treating a nosebleed which comes from a rupture of blood vessels in Kiesselbach's triangle?
    A. have child in a sitting position with head slightly tilted back
    B. compress both nostrils between fingers for no less than ten minutes
    C. release and compress intermittently to check on blood stoppage
    D. place ice pack over bridge of nose or against nape of neck (1:93)

56. In examining the fontanels, the nurse should direct her attention to
    A. size, pulsations, tenseness, number and position
    B. condition of anterior and posterior fontanels
    C. appearance and any sign of dehydration
    D. A and B (1:40)

57. Which of the following conditions lead to late closure of fontanels?

A. cretinism, syphilis, Down's syndrome
   B. microcephaly, scurvy, kwashiorkor
   C. normocephaly, hydrocephaly, Waardenburg's syndrome
   D. A and C (1:40)

58. Definite great pulsations of the fontanels may be an indication of what condition?
    A. dehydration
    B. hypoglycemia
    C. intracranial pressure
    D. hyperglycemia (1:40)

59. The occipital lymph nodes should not be palpable in the following conditions, except in
    A. encephalitis
    B. roseola infantum or rubella
    C. meningitis
    D. none of the above (1:41)

60. Children with a white streak of hair running from their forehead towards the crown of their head may have Waardenburg's syndrome and should be inspected for
    A. kwashiorkor — reddish
    B. syphilis
    C. deafness
    D. vitamin A deficiency (1:41)

61. Normal hair should show the following characteristics, except
    A. smooth, fine texture
    B. even distribution over the scalp
    C. coarse, dry texture
    D. A and B (1:41)

62. Head control is attained gradually, but should be almost complete by
    A. five months
    B. three months
    C. nine months
    D. twelve months (1:41)

63. Which of the following signs is most often associated with mental retardation or kidney abnormalities?
    A. pinna of ears crossing or touching eye-occiput line
    B. pinna of ears crossing below eye-occiput line
    C. marked decrease in chin
    D. circumoral cyanosis (1:42)

64. Excessive pulsations observed and palpated in the neck may be signs of
    A. cardiac problems
    B. respiratory arrest
    C. kidney abnormalities
    D. hypertelorism (1:43)

65. Craniotabes, the softening of the outer layer of the skull, will display a ping-pong snapping sensation if scalp is
    A. firmly pressed along coronal suture
    B. firmly pressed over the occipital bones just below the coronal sutures
    C. firmly pressed behind and above ears in temporoparietal region and along suture
    D. firmly pressed along sagittal sutures (1:43)

66. You are examining an infant's head and discover that one side of the occipital area is decidedly flat. Which of the following factors might be irrelevant to the condition?
    A. crib is placed against a certain wall
    B. infant is always placed in crib the same way
    C. infant always prefers to lie on that side
    D. child is made to sit up more often (1:44)

The Eyes

Directions: Match the following numbered items with the most appropriate lettered items.

E 67. Excessive blinking (1:54)
H 68. Edema of conjunctiva (1:57)
A 69. Excessive tearing (1:51)
B 70. Dropping of upper eyelid (1:54)
C 71. Light or white speckling of outer two-thirds of iris (1:62)
L 72. Continuous jerky movement of iris and pupil (1:62)
D 73. Clouding of lens (1:63)
G 74. Irregular yellow patches on palpebral conjunctiva, signs of vitamin A deficiency (1:58)

Health Maintenance and Promotion

75. Inflammation of meibomian glands (1:55)
76. Infection of lacrimal system (1:57)

    A. Epiphora
    B. Ptosis
    C. Brushfield's spots
    D. Cataract
    E. Blepharospasm
    F. Cornea
    G. Bitol's spots
    H. Chemosis
    I. Stye
    J. Dacryoadenitis
    K. Dacryocystitis
    L. Nystagmus

Directions: For each of the following multiple choice questions, select the ONE most appropriate answer.

77. The thick, tough, opaque, inelastic membrane covering about five-sixths of the eye is the
    A. sclera
    B. cornea
    C. iris
    D. retina (1:51)

78. The vascular layer of the eye is composed of the following, except the
    A. choroid
    B. ciliary body
    C. retina
    D. iris (1:52)

79. Vision is most perfect in the
    A. macula
    B. fovea centralis
    C. optic disc
    D. pars ciliaris retinae (1:52)

80. Which of the following is not a structure of refraction within the eye proper?
    A. aqueous humor
    B. cornea
    C. optic disc
    D. vitreous body (1:53)

81. Which of the following techniques is *not* generally used in evaluating the eye?
    A. inspection
    B. palpation
    C. auscultation
    D. percussion (1:53)

82. The child's automatic raising of the opposite eyelid when his jaw is moved to one side reveals the
    A. Marcus Gunn reflex
    B. Babinsky reflex
    C. Kernig's reflex
    D. Chadwick's sign (1:54)

83. The condition in which the eyelids do not close entirely, resulting from facial nerve paralysis or congenitally shortened muscles is called
    A. exophthalmus
    B. Horner's syndrome
    C. lagophthalmus
    D. Treacher Collins syndrome (1:54)

84. Eyelashes are particularly bushy in
    A. Treacher Collins disease
    B. premature infants
    C. Down's syndrome
    D. Hurler's syndrome (1:57)

85. A condition in which tears are produced in inadequate amounts is called
    A. dysautonomia
    B. epiphora
    C. chemosis
    D. dacryo-adenitis (1:57)

86. A test which should be performed on every child over six months of age, to rule out subtle strabismus, is the
    A. Romberg's test
    B. Hirschberg test
    C. Snellen test
    D. Ishihur test (1:59)

The Skeletal, Integumentary, and Lymphatic System

Directions: Match the following numbered items with the most appropriate lettered items.

87. Fusion or webbing of 2 or more phalanges (1:202)
88. Movement away from the medial line (1:191)

89. Upper portion of hip bone (1:195) — G
90. Knock-knees (1:204) — B
91. A very high arch of foot (1:205) — F
92. Toeing out (1:206) — A
93. Stabilization of joint that should be movable (1:210) — E
94. Extra digits on hands or feet (1:202) — D
95. Bowleggedness (1:203) — L
96. Exaggerated convex curve in lumbar region of spine (1:207) — C

   A. Pes valgus
   B. Genu valgum
   C. Lordosis
   D. Polydactyly
   E. Ankylosis
   F. Pes cavus
   G. Ilium
   H. Abduction
   I. Syndactyly
   J. Ischium
   K. Kyphosis
   L. Genu varus

Directions: For each of the following multiple choice questions, select the ONE most appropriate answer.

97. All of the following are functions of the skin, except
    A. protecting deeper tissues from injury, drying, and foreign matter invasion
    B. regulating body temperature
    C. providing for excretion
    D. production of vitamin K (1:10)

98. The nonvascular part of the skin is called
    A. dermis
    B. epidermis
    C. stratum granulosum
    D. stratum lucidum (1:11)

99. Which part of the skin accounts for the black, brown and tawny colors of the different races?
    A. stratum corneum
    B. stratum lucidum
    C. stratum spinosum
    D. stratum basale (1:11)

100. Hair growth is cyclic. Which stage is **the** transition between activity and nonactivity?
    A. anagen
    B. catagen
    C. gelogen
    D. none of the above (1:13)

101. Physiologic jaundice appears about 24 hours after birth and disappears by the
    A. first week
    B. second week
    C. third week
    D. fourth week (1:15)

102. Erythroblastosis fetalis causes jaundice at birth or within the first
    A. 24 hours
    B. 16 hours
    C. 12 hours
    D. 48 hours (1:15)

103. The infant with a beefy-red color over his entire body may be suffering from
    A. anemia
    B. leukemia
    C. polycythemia
    D. hypoglycemia (1:15)

104. A test for skin turgor is best done by
    A. tapping skin on lower abdomen
    B. taking a large pinch of skin on lower abdomen
    C. feeling calf of leg
    D. B and C (1:15)

105. Rough and dry skin may be caused by all of the following, except
    A. frequent bathing
    B. cold weather
    C. vitamin C deficiency
    D. hypothyroidism (1:16)

106. Scaliness over the scalp, spreading to **a** red macular rash over the forehead, cheeks, neck and chest can be seborrhea and usually clears with
    A. application of baby powder
    B. application of baby oil
    C. washing with plain soap and water
    D. penicillin ointment (1:16)

Health Maintenance and Promotion

107. The tiny, red, irritated lesions found in prickly heat are called
    A. milia
    B. hemangiomas
    C. xanthomas
    D. erythemas (1:17)

108. The best way to clear up the aforenoted condition is to
    A. apply talcum powder all over baby's body
    B. keep baby cool with less restrictive bedding and clothing
    C. bathe baby with pHisoHex® solution
    D. bathe baby with thin cornstarch solution (1:17)

109. Another name for nevus flammeus is
    A. strawberry mark
    B. cavernous hemangioma
    C. port wine stain
    D. cafe-au-lait spots (1:18)

110. Trauma to the skin produces ecchymosis. Under what conditions would ecchymosis be of great concern to the nurse?
    A. when observed all over the child's body, with a history of decreased play and activity
    B. when markedly observed below the knees and elbows, with a history of rough games and increased activity
    C. when displayed in peculiar places, with a history of odd and unusual falls or accidents
    D. A and C (1:18)

Directions: Match the following numbered items with the most appropriate lettered items.

111. Soft, reddish, rounded lesions present at birth (1:18)
112. Bacterial infection causing formation of painful nodule around hair follicle or sweat gland (1:55)
113. Normal fullness and resistance seen in healthy skin (1:15)
114. Flat, small lesion which shows a color change (1:18)
115. First fine hairs covering body during fetal life (1:13,20)
116. Elevated, sharply circumscribed lesion filled with pus (1:19)
117. Cheesy, white material covering entire body of some newborns (1:13)
118. Absence of pigment in skin (1:15)
119. Small yellow plaques seen across the nose of many newborns (1:17)
120. Itching condition (1:32)

   A. Macule
   B. Scales
   C. Pruritus
   D. Vernix caseosa
   E. Pustule
   F. Lanugo
   G. Wheal
   H. Cavernous hemangiomas
   I. Turgor
   J. Vitiligo
   K. Xanthomas
   L. Seborrhea
   M. Furuncles

Directions: For each of the following multiple choice questions, select the ONE most appropriate answer.

121. An elevated white-to-pink edematous lesion associated with pruritus is called
    A. vesicle
    B. erosion
    C. wheal
    D. papule (1:19)

122. A condition where the epidermis is mechanically removed, leaving the dermis exposed, best describes
    A. crusts
    B. excoriation
    C. erosion
    D. lichenification (1:19)

123. A sharply defined lesion filled with clean free fluid is called a
    A. vesicle
    B. wheal
    C. papule
    D. macule (1:19)

124. An increase and thickening of the epidermis and dermis is termed
    A. scars
    B. bullae
    C. ulcers
    D. lichenification (1:19)

125. Which of the following characteristics best describe a papule?
    A. flat, sharply circumscribed, big, lightly colored lesion
    B. flat, sharply circumscribed, small and colored lesion
    C. elevated, sharply circumscribed lesion filled with pus
    D. elevated, sharply circumscribed lesion filled with clear fluid (1:18)

126. Sores resulting from destruction and loss of epidermis, dermis, and possibly subcutaneous layers are commonly known as
    A. excoriations
    B. erosions
    C. ulcers
    D. pustules (1:19)

127. Normal newborns begin to sweat
    A. soon after birth
    B. when they are about one month old
    C. when they are about two months old
    D. when they are about three months old (1:19)

128. The most essential equipment in the examination of the skin is a
    A. flashlight
    B. good source of natural lighting
    C. Wood's lamp
    D. none of the above (1:21)

129. In examining the skin, the nurse must rely heavily on her techniques of the following, except
    A. percussion
    B. palpation
    C. inspection
    D. observation (1:21)

130. A young mother asks you what to do with her baby who is moderately covered with miliaria. Your advice should include
    A. dress your baby comfortably in a cotton shirt or nightie and diaper
    B. never use wool directly over his skin
    C. adjust room temperature to 70° F
    D. all of the above (1:21)

131. Your advice to a mother whose baby shows a marked "cradle cap" should include the following, except
    A. washing the scalp daily, using soap and firm pressure, even over the fontanel
    B. rinsing the scalp thoroughly after soaping
    C. applying oil to the scalp *after* the bath
    D. applying a small amount of oil to the scalp, massaging it in, and combing the hair with a fine baby comb *before* the bath (1:122)

132. Which of the following conditions favors the occurrence of ammoniacal diaper rash in infants?
    A. frequent diaper change
    B. using tight-fitting diapers and plastic pants
    C. rinsing of buttocks and genitalia before diaper change
    D. applying baby powder during diaper change (1:22)

133. Treatment for mild diaper rash in infants is facilitated by
    A. leaving diaper off during nap time
    B. turning infant on his abdomen, placing diaper under buttock area, and leaving buttocks exposed
    C. applying thin layer of petrolatum jelly or A & D ointment after each diaper change and vigorously removing with each cleaning
    D. all of the above (1:23)

134. Prevention of diaper rash centers primarily on
    A. care of diapers
    B. care of baby
    C. care of mother
    D. A and B (1:23)

135. Which of the following is not a lymphatic organ?
    A. tonsils

Health Maintenance and Promotion

B. stomach
C. spleen
D. thymus (1:26)

136. The greatest number of palpable nodes are concentrated in the
A. axillae
B. anus
C. head
D. groin (1:27)

137. Normal nodes are characterized as
A. nontender and cool
B. "fixed" or "immobile"
C. easily moved under the fingers during palpation
D. A and C (1:27)

138. Which nodes are enlarged in the presence of foot and leg infections?
A. submental nodes
B. inguinal nodes
C. axillary nodes
D. epitrochlear nodes (1:27)

139. Tick bites can cause which nodes to swell?
A. occipital
B. superficial cervical
C. submental
D. parotid (1:27)

140. The areas which should be examined for lymph nodes during every physical examination are the following, except
A. head and neck
B. axillary and arm
C. breast
D. inguinal (1:28)

141. Small firm nodes are called
A. "shotty"
B. telangiectasis
C. adenopathy
D. petechia (1:29)

The Respiratory System

Directions: Match the following numbered items with the most appropriate lettered items.

C 142. Difficult breathing (1:123)
I 143. Lateral curvature of the spine (1:207)
L 144. Crackling sound caused by the escape of air into the subcutaneous fat (1:160)
F 145. Slow breathing (1:121)
A 146. Deep breathing characteristic of metabolic acidosis (1:123)
B 147. Total amount of air that can be expelled after a full inspiration (1:117)
H 148. Rapid irregular breathing, first shallow and then deep (1:123)
G 149. Regular, predictable pattern of several breaths followed by a pause and again by several breaths (1:123)
E 150. Exaggerated concave curve in the thoracic region (1:119)
J 151. Exchange of gases from air into bloodstream and vice versa (1:117)

A. Kussmaul breathing
B. Vital capacity
C. Dyspnea
D. Cogwheel breath sounds
E. Kyphosis
F. Bradypnea
G. Cheyne-Stokes respiration
H. Biots' breathing
I. Scoliosis
J. Respiration
K. Tidal air
L. Crepitation

Directions: For each of the following multiple choice questions, select the ONE most appropriate answer.

152. Which of the following structures separates the abdominal cavity from the thoracic cavity?
A. diaphragm
B. sternum
C. thorax
D. sternocleidomastoid muscles (1:113)

153. The chest cavity is divided into halves, with the middle portion known as the
A. pleura
B. mediastinum
C. areola
D. bronchioles (1:116)

154. The membrane that covers the diaphragm and inner surface of the chest wall is called the
A. pulmonary pleura

B. mediastinum
C. parietal pleura
D. peritoneum (1:116)

155. Which of the following structures is known as the voice box?
A. pharynx
B. trachea
C. esophagus
D. larynx (1:116)

156. Which of the following signs is indicative of vitamin C deficiency?
A. kyphosis
B. scoliosis
C. lordosis
D. rachitic rosary (1:119)

157. Which of the following signs may indicate pulmonary emphysema or asthma or cystic fibrosis?
A. funnel breast
B. barrel chest
C. Harrison's groove
D. gibbus (1:119)

158. Concerning adolescent respiration rate, the normal range of inspirations per minute is
A. 40–60
B. 30–40
C. 20–30
D. 10–20 (1:121)

159. Respiration in infancy is characteristically
A. abdominal
B. costal
C. tachypneic
D. bradypneic (1:122)

160. Breath sounds should always be evaluated as to
A. pitch
B. intensity and duration
C. quality
D. all of the above (1:124,125)

The Cardiovascular System

Directions: Match the following numbered items with the most appropriate lettered items.

161. Slow pulse (1:140)
162. Muscular layer of the heart (1:132)
163. First heart sound caused by the contraction of the ventricles (1:139)
164. Heart murmur indicating an underlying pathologic condition (1:142)
165. Transmits impulses controlling the heartbeat (1:147)
166. Classic area for auscultation of the heart, located at the third, fourth and fifth intercostal spaces (1:138)
167. Very irregular rhythm caused by rapid, uncoordinated contracting of atria (1:140)
168. Forceful bounding pulse, best felt at radial and femoral areas and accompanied by increase in pulse pressure (1:130)
169. Classic area for auscultation of the heart, located in the second and third left intercostal space, near the sternum (1:142)
170. Abnormal heart sound similar to a click, often due to mitral stenosis (1:141)

A. Organic murmur
B. Systole
C. Precordial area
D. Opening snap
E. Myocardium
F. Pulmonic area
G. Functional murmur
H. Bradycardia
I. Water-hammer pulse
J. Bundle of His
K. Pericardium
L. Atrial fibrillation

Directions: For each of the following multiple choice questions, select the ONE most appropriate answer.

171. Which of the following causes the highest incidence of morbidity and mortality in infancy?
A. rheumatic fever
B. congenital heart defects
C. infections
D. accidents (1:131)

172. The second largest cause of cardiac problems in the pediatric age group is
A. rheumatic fever
B. tetralogy of fallot
C. pulmonary atresia
D. coarctation of the aorta (1:131)

Health Maintenance and Promotion

173. The normal pulse rate for preschoolers ranges from
    A. 70–170/min
    B. 80–160/min
    C. 80–120/min
    D. 70–100/min   (1:134)

174. Which of the following conditions is *not* associated with an increase in pulse rate?
    A. excitement
    B. severe anemia
    C. Salmonella infection
    D. none of the above   (1:134)

175. The difference between systolic and diastolic readings is called
    A. systolic pressure
    B. pulse pressure
    C. diastolic pressure
    D. Corrigan's pulse   (1:136)

176. Which of the following statements is accurate about blood pressure readings?
    A. an abnormally low diastolic reading is usually more important than an abnormally high systolic reading
    B. an unusually high systolic reading may indicate patent ductus arteriosus, exercise or excitement
    C. an abnormally low diastolic reading may indicate fever, aortic regurgitation or aortic stenosis
    D. aortic stenosis may be reflected in an abnormally wide pulse pressure   (1:136)

177. The first heart sound (S₁) is caused by the closure of the
    A. mitral valve
    B. semilunar valves
    C. tricuspid valves
    D. A and C   (1:139)

The Abdomen

Directions: Match the following numbered items with the most appropriate lettered items.

178. Sphincter of the stomach through which food passes from the esophagus   (1:151)
179. Bluish umbilicus resulting from intra-abdominal hemorrhage   (1:156)
180. The shortest, most immobile portion of the small intestine   (1:152)
181. Enlarged palpable organs   (1:149,155)
182. An accumulation of serous fluid in the abdomen   (1:155,156)
183. A sign of liver disease   (1:156)
184. A very dilated, hypotonic colon usually with very little peristalsis   (1:155)
185. A massive ecchymosis, usually on flanks and lower abdomen indicating extravasation of blood from within the abdomen   (1:156)
186. "Stretch marks"   (1:156)
187. Muscular defect which allows internal organs to protrude   (1:157)

    A. Megacolon
    B. Grey Turner's sign
    C. Spider nevi
    D. Ascites
    E. Striae
    F. Cardiac valve
    G. Hernia
    H. Cullen's sign
    I. Paralytic ileus
    J. Organomegaly
    K. Pylorus
    L. Duodenum

Directions: For each of the following multiple choice questions, select the ONE most appropriate answer.

188. Food moves through the stomach into the intestine by means of
    A. peristalsis
    B. constant pressure
    C. gravitational push
    D. osmosis   (1:151)

189. Which part of the small intestine is vascular and contains large villi?
    A. duodenum
    B. jejunum
    C. ileum
    D. A and C   (1:152)

190. Which one is the largest and heaviest gland in the body?

A. pancreas
B. stomach
C. spleen
D. liver (1:152)

191. The main functions of the liver are the following, except
A. production of bile
B. metabolism of proteins and carbohydrates
C. secretion of insulin
D. aids in development of red blood cells (1:152,153)

192. Which organ helps with the production of red blood cells during the first year of life, but thereafter aids in the destruction of red blood cells?
A. liver
B. spleen
C. pancreas
D. gallbladder (1:153)

193. Which of the following is the classic sign of pyloric stenosis?
A. projectile vomiting
B. abdominal distention
C. peristaltic waves which move from left to right
D. paradoxical respiration (1:155)

194. Which of the following changes in the umbilicus may be a sign of abdominal cancer?
A. bluish umbilicus
B. nodular umbilicus
C. everted umbilicus
D. sunken umbilicus (1:156)

195. Which of the following statements is *not* true of umbilical hernias?
A. umbilical hernias ordinarily attain their maximum size by 1 year of age and generally close by 6 years of age
B. umbilical hernias ordinarily attain their maximum size by 1 month of age and generally close by 1 year of age
C. size of umbilical hernia should always be judged by palpating actual opening, not by measuring contents protruding through opening
D. taping a coin into umbilical ring can interfere with its closure, and therefore such practice should never be done (1:157)

196. Which of the following conditions of the umbilicus of newborns does not necessarily call for immediate intervention?
A. foul-smelling discharge from umbilicus
B. periumbilical redness and induration
C. skin warmth
D. bulging of umbilical area (1:156)

197. Excessive hairiness on the abdomen of infants and children may be a sign of
A. childhood diabetes
B. transexuality
C. adrenal-cortical problems
D. liver disorders (1:156)

198. Which of the following is true about femoral hernia?
A. it is a congenital condition
B. it is more common in females than males
C. it presents as a bulge through the wall of inguinal canal in femoral area
D. it is much more frequent in males than females (1:158)

199. A murmur heard near the umbilical area is suggestive of
A. renal artery defect
B. congenital abnormalities of umbilical vein
C. ascites
D. inflamed spleen (1:159)

200. Accurate assessment of a child's abdomen by palpation is best achieved by observing the following guidelines, except
A. keeping examiner's hands warm
B. placing a pillow beneath child's head
C. flexing child's knees
D. employing a firm, forceful touch (1:159)

Neurologic Examination

201. The central nervous system contains the
A. encephalon and medulla spinalis

B. encephalon and medulla oblongata
C. diencephalon and mesencephalon
D. diencephalon and telencephalon (1:213)

202. Groups of nerves found outside the central nervous system are called
A. neurons
B. axons
C. ganglia
D. dendrites (1:213)

203. Which of the following structures is called gray matter?
A. meninges
B. cortex
C. dura matter
D. pia matter (1:213,214)

204. A spinal puncture in the lumbar region enters the
A. subdural area between the third and fourth lumbar vertebrae
B. subarachnoid area between the second and third lumbar vertebrae
C. subdural area between the second and third lumbar vertebrae
D. subarachnoid area between the third and fourth lumbar vertebrae (13:251)

205. Motor aphasia can result from damage to
A. Broca's area
B. precentral cortex
C. premotor area
D. A and B (1:144)

206. Deep pressure pain can be tested in any of the following areas, *except* the
A. testes
B. Achilles tendon
C. abdominal muscles
D. calf and forearm muscles (1:240)

207. Excessive drowsiness in an infant or young child may indicate the following conditions, *except*
A. metabolic problem
B. hypothalamic disease
C. diffuse brain tumor
D. severe avitaminosis (1:221)

208. If a child is asked what he had for dinner last night and tells you every item, you recognize his response as reflective of good
A. remote memory
B. recent memory
C. immediate recall
D. confabulation (1:222)

209. The ability to perceive weight or direction of movement is called
A. graphesthesia
B. stereogenesis
C. kinesthesia
D. alexia (1:223)

210. Stereogenesis is best described as the ability to
A. identify shapes traced by examiner on palm or back of child's hand
B. recognize an object from its feel
C. perceive weight or direction of movement
D. identify sounds when child's eyes are closed (1:222,223)

211. The child's directional sense is tested by playing games, such as
A. the "up-down game"
B. the "rough-smooth game"
C. "hide and seek"
D. A and C (1:223)

212. Whereas problems of visual agnosia usually originate in the occipital lobe, tactile agnosia originates in the
A. lateral temporal lobe
B. superior portion of temporal lobe
C. parietal lobe
D. postero-inferior areas of parietal lobe (1:223)

213. Testing for the first cranial nerve (olfactory nerve) is concerned with the sense of
A. taste
B. sight
C. pressure
D. smell (1:255)

214. Which of the following cranial nerves has both a sensory and motor division?

A. olfactory and optic nerves
B. optic and facial nerves
C. facial and trigeminal nerves
D. trigeminal and optic nerves
(1:226,227)

215. Which area of the brain primarily controls balance and coordination?
A. cerebrum
B. cerebellum
C. pons
D. medulla oblongata (1:230)

216. Which of the following can be used to test for cerebellar function?
A. have child walk in his normal gait with his eyes open, then closed, and finally walking tandem
B. have child "make a face"
C. have child identify shapes traced by examiner on palm of child's hand
D. have child repeat sounds after examiner (1:232)

217. A nurse should know that for the first two months an infant's muscle tone is expected to be primarily *what* type?
A. extensor
B. abductor
C. adductor
D. flexor (1:236)

218. As the child enters the stage of extension, *what* may begin to appear in the case of an infant with cerebral palsy?
A. tonicity
B. spasticity
C. clonicity
D. flexibility (1:236)

219. When the examiner pushes the infant's head forward, a child with beginning signs of cerebral palsy will
A. frequently flex his neck with examiner's hand
B. hardly resist pressure and readily flex his neck with examiner's hand
C. frequently resist presssure and extend his neck back against examiner's hand
D. readily extend and adduct his legs, perhaps even crossing (1:236)

220. The normal posture of a newborn is generally one of
A. symmetry with limbs semiflexed and hips slightly abducted
B. asymmetry with one limb semiflexed and hips slightly abducted
C. symmetry with limbs extended and hips markedly abducted
D. asymmetry with one limb semiflexed and hips markedly abducted (1:237)

221. There are several abnormal postures which should serve as red flags to the examiner. Which of the following is *not always* a cause of concern?
A. opisthotonus
B. undue rotation of head
C. a hand held constantly over head
D. frog position (1:237)

222. A full-term infant should be expected to
A. hold his head at a 45° angle or less from horizontal line
B. hold back straight or slightly flexed
C. assume arms flexed at elbows and partially extended at shoulders
D. all of the above (1:237)

223. Slow, worm-like, irregular movements may be a sign of
A. extrapyramidal syndromes
B. athetoid cerebral palsy
C. Down's syndrome
D. cri-du-chat syndrome (1:239)

224. The brachioradialis reflex is initiated by a sharp tap of the reflex hammer to the styloid process of the radius resulting in
A. flexion of elbow and pronation of forearm
B. flexion of knee with kicking action
C. contraction of triceps thus extending elbow
D. plantar flexion of foot (1:244)

225. Which reflex is tested by stroking the lateral aspect of the sole of the foot with a relatively sharp object, such as a pinpoint or fingernail?
A. Moro reflex
B. Achilles reflex

C. Babinski reflex
D. Kernig's reflex (1:245,246)

226. Which type of reflex is abnormal *only* after the child has begun to walk?
A. Moro reflex
B. Achilles reflex
C. Babinski reflex
D. Kernig's reflex (1:246)

227. The reflex that is elicited by stroking the lateral aspect of the foot directly under the lateral malleolus is called
A. Chaddock reflex
B. Oppenheim reflex
C. Gordon reflex
D. Achilles reflex (1:246,247)

228. The tonic neck reflex has its peak incidence at about
A. two to three months
B. four to five months
C. six to seven months
D. one to two months (1:247)

229. The tonic neck reflex should be considered abnormal past how many months?
A. eight
B. six
C. ten
D. twelve (1:247)

230. Which of the following techniques elicits the rooting reflex?
A. touch corners or middle of upper or lower lip of infant
B. prick sole of infant's foot with pin
C. apply light pressure to soles of infant's feet
D. press thumbs sharply against soles of infant's feet (1:249)

231. Sucking is vital to an infant's life, and it should be observed for
A. strength of tongue action
B. rate
C. pattern of grouping in the suck
D. all of the above (1:251)

232. The most important reflex in the young infant (and should always be tested) is probably the
A. Chaddock reflex
B. Babinski reflex
C. Moro reflex
D. patellar reflex (1:251)

Directions: Match the following numbered items with the most appropriate lettered items.

233. Concerned with circulation and respiration (1:217)
234. Involved with temperature control, water balance, and some digestive activities (1:216)
235. Functions in transition of sensory impulses to cortex (1:216)
236. Awareness of one's own bodily posture and movement (1:216)
237. Basic unit of the nervous system (1:212,213)
238. Serves as a neural transmission center (1:216)
239. Involved in controlling ability to articulate speech (1:214)
240. Receives impulses and transmits them to cell body (1:213)
241. Transmits impulses from cell body outward to rest of body (1:213)
242. Involved in integrating several types of stimulation from various sensory areas (1:215)

A. Proprioception
B. Pons
C. Hypothalamus
D. Medulla oblongata
E. Neuron
F. Broca's area
G. Axon
H. Thalamus
I. Parietal area
J. Dendrite
K. Encephalon

B. Psychosocial Assessments

Directions: For each of the following multiple choice questions, select the ONE most appropriate answer.

243. Anxiety plays an important role in normal development. It is best described as a (an)

A. feeling of apprehension and tension of a particularly disturbing nature produced by both external and internal danger
B. specific feeling of dread associated with a pounding heart
C. signal that the individual is losing his mind
D. intense feeling of apprehension associated with a specific object (10:339)

244. Anxiety primarily differs from fear in that the former
A. occurs when satisfaction of physiological needs is deferred
B. clarifies factors prevailing in current situation
C. is acquired by empathic linkage
D. is associated mostly with authority figures (27:87,92)

245. The nursing intervention for a child with anxiety demands that the nurse do the following *except*
A. take his complaints at face value
B. treat his complaints objectively while retaining her perception for child's subtle needs
C. place psychological implications on every complaint
D. help him identify and deal with those things that worry him (24:92)

246. A child who breaks a toy when asked to return it to the owner is best described as
A. frustrated
B. anxious
C. aggressive
D. regressive (24:97)

247. Which of the following statements is true about aggression in children?
A. aggression is always associated with hostility
B. children's aggression is primarily a covert behavior
C. degree of intensity in the expression of a child's aggression does not correlate with his hostility
D. aggression in children may be seen in terms of group leadership (24:97)

248. Helping the aggressive child is primarily aimed at
A. destroying his aggression
B. aiding him to direct his aggression into useful channels in life
C. reinforcing his aggressive behavior so that he will feel recognized
D. easing parental problems in dealing with child (24:98,99)

249. Which of the following is *not* seen as a therapeutic purpose of play?
A. safety valve for pent-up instinctual drives
B. supports fantasy of strength
C. helps child deal actively with painful situations
D. denies terrifying as well as gratifying experiences (13:534)

250. Which of the following is *least* helpful in releasing aggressive feelings?
A. bean bag throws
B. punching clown
C. musical toy
D. pounding board (24:97,98)

251. The anxiety that appears in anticipation of a danger situation is referred to as
A. traumatic anxiety
B. artificial anxiety
C. signal anxiety
D. natural anxiety (10:339)

252. Which of the following behaviors could be least expected in an anxious child?
A. excessively quiet and withdrawn
B. fretful
C. worried
D. disrupting conversation (27:92)

253. Which of the following mechanisms would serve as a rich resource for children experiencing fear and anxiety?
A. withdrawal
B. displacement
C. acting-out
D. B and C (24:95)

254. A child who attacks whatever is within reach or whomever is near is best described as displaying

A. aggression
B. diffuse aggression
C. regression
D. rebellion (24:97)

255. Which of the following mechanisms is *most* likely adopted by a child experiencing an overwhelming sense of guilt?
A. repression
B. aggression
C. regression
D. isolation (24:95)

256. Which of the following mechanisms would be *least* likely adopted by children confronted with situations of reality-determined fears?
A. sharpening their reality testing to be more vigilant in the future
B. learning to avoid the danger, without having to leave the danger-involving activity
C. clinging to fantasies of power, force, and indestructibility
D. unconditional direct confrontation (24:94)

257. When a child abandons a given activity in panic and continues to avoid this otherwise pleasure-promising activity, the nurse should recognize the behavior as
A. withdrawal
B. total flight and avoidance
C. regression
D. dependency (24:96)

258. According to Erikson's stages of personality development, the toddler's (age 1–3) major psychosocial task is to develop
A. autonomy
B. identity
C. trust
D. initiative (13:417)

259. During the toddler period, children generally preface most conversations with
A. "why?"
B. "no"
C. "me"
D. "I" (13:419)

260. Which of the following best describes a healthy three-year-old?
A. grows rapidly, feeds self, names figures in a picture
B. helps dress himself, attempts to sing songs, talks in complete sentences
C. sits quietly at the table, has a vocabulary of approximately 900 words, goes on errands outside the home
D. is toilet trained at night, understands time, participates in imaginative play (13:434)

261. A mother describes her son as not being interested in playing with other children. "He doesn't fight with them, but simply ignores them and plays by himself in the same room." Your *best* response about her two-year-old would be
A. "As long as they don't fight, don't worry about it."
B. "Toddlers seldom play with other children, but enjoy playing in the same room."
C. "Children this age are inconsistent in play patterns. Don't worry about it."
D. "This is called parallel play and is a bit advanced for your son." (13:434)

262. A nurse hears a child say, "The kids at school don't like me very good because my clothes aren't nice and my house isn't good." What should the nurse do in this situation?
A. respond with an understanding of his feeling
B. send a referral to social service
C. find ways to increase his self-esteem
D. nothing, as this is something she can do nothing about (13:602)

263. Danger signals that should make a nurse think of disturbed interpersonal relations in an older child are the following, except
A. failure to discriminate adequately between familiar and unfamiliar people
B. difficulties in playing with others at a level expected of his age
C. constriction of range and repertoire of positive and negative feelings
D. none of the above (27:100)

264. Timmy, age four, began to exhibit personality deviations as a result of the return of his father, a Vietnam veteran. The return of his father could be an example of
   A. accession
   B. direct aggression
   C. identity diffusion
   D. demoralization (13:523,524)

265. An adolescent is taking an interest in religion. You should recognize this as
   A. normal for this age group
   B. an expression of fear
   C. a sign of guilt
   D. a sign of rebellion (13:684)

266. Freud, Erikson and Piaget have formulated theories of personality development. Which of the following stages of development fits the theories for preschoolers?
   A. genital stage, initiative vs. guilt and intuitive phase
   B. latent stage, industry vs. inferiority and preconceptual stage
   C. genital stage, identity vs. identity and concrete operations
   D. anal stage, trust vs. mistrust and preconceptual stage (13:515,516)

267. Johnny is approximately three years old and is, according to Erikson, beginning to accept reality versus the pleasure principle, which relates to which of the following psychosocial crises?
   A. identity vs. identity diffusion
   B. initiative vs. guilt
   C. autonomy vs. shame and doubt
   D. industry vs. inferiority (9:253)

268. An eight-year-old boy was hospitalized due to problems with his diabetic diet. When questioning *him* in the presence of his mother about his diet at home, the nurse was answered always by his mother. This is an example of
   A. gate-keeping
   B. status
   C. triangling
   D. reaction formation (13:630,631)

269. Which of the following is a true statement about crisis?
   A. after the initial impact, periods of recoil and trauma can still be avoided
   B. reorganization levels are always reached following crisis
   C. the crisis does not need to be perceived as such by the family for crisis to occur
   D. unresolved key problems are repressed until after resolution of the crisis (13:681,682)

270. While the healthy adolescent is establishing his sense of intimacy, he has a real struggle with
   A. parental emancipation
   B. sexual feelings
   C. peer acceptance
   D. self reliance (13:683)

271. Which of the following is *not* common in the development of prejudice in individuals?
   A. need for categorization
   B. group solidarity in the individual's own group
   C. scapegoating aggression stemming from frustration
   D. open relatedness with members of other groups (13:127,128,129)

272. Environmental deprivation is best described as
   A. total absence of mothering
   B. a complicated process with multiple causes
   C. any external event or constellation of events which significantly interferes with a child's normal developmental processes, thus affecting adversely his mental or physical status
   D. intentional withholding of something essential for healthy personality development (10:275)

273. In America, the chief environmental factor for the development of the child is represented by the
   A. family
   B. school

C. church
D. social clubs (10:275,276)

274. Studies of the impact of deprivation upon the development of children have been greatly attributed to the works of
   A. Bowlby
   B. Spitz
   C. Glueck
   D. A and B (10:277)

275. Clinical manifestations seen in infants deprived of adequate mothering may include the following, *except*
   A. poor appetite and excessive weeping
   B. excessive thumb-sucking and emotional affect
   C. emaciation and failure to thrive
   D. excessive rocking and retardation of speech (10:277)

276. Anaclitic depression follows which of the following sequences of responses?
   A. protest to denial to despair
   B. denial to protest to despair
   C. protest to despair to denial
   D. despair to protest to denial (13:301)

277. Which of the following groups of children is seen to be most devastatingly affected by deprivation?
   A. children less than 1 year of age
   B. children less than 30 months of age
   C. children from 3 to 4 years of age
   D. children from 4 to 6 years of age (10:278)

278. Prevention of maternal deprivation should basically
   A. involve early detection and special attention to the children from high-risk categories
   B. expand foster care and institutional facilities
   C. provide for early adoptions
   D. improve total school milieu (10:279)

279. Under what conditions is anxiety considered pathologic?
   A. when it is much greater or persists much longer than is appropriate for the situation
   B. when it does not respond to realistic reassurance
   C. when it is so severe as to be paralyzing
   D. all of the above (10:339)

280. Which of the following statements does *not* reflect the nature of traumatic anxiety?
   A. it develops automatically when the influx of stimuli is too overwhelming for the child to cope
   B. it plays a great role in normal development
   C. its prototype is birth
   D. it is characteristic of infancy because of the immaturity of the ego at that time of life (10:339)

281. Bobby was placed in a foundling home shortly after birth. Because of a high ratio of children to staff members, and low sensory stimulation received, at 4 months of age he exhibited signs of maternal deprivation. Which of the following characteristics would not relate to maternal deprivation?
   A. loss of weight
   B. seeking contact with adults
   C. poor resistance to infection
   D. retarded motor development (10:278)

282. Which of the following nursing measures is *least* effective in meeting an infant's need for sensory stimulation?
   A. periodic change in position and rhythmic rocking
   B. exposing him to various textures of materials and sounds
   C. placing him continuously in playpen decorated with mobiles
   D. talking and singing to him while being cuddled (13:282)

283. Weaning of an infant should *never* be undertaken under which of the following conditions?
   A. he has not yet demonstrated the ability to drink well from the cup
   B. sibling is hospitalized for rheumatic fever

C. mother is pregnant
D.) infant is sick and hospitalized
(13:314)

284. Children having an unusually low frustration threshold are best described as
   A. not allowing themselves to be frustrated but insisting upon a total gratification of all eminent impulses
   B. extremely withdrawn, anxious, rebellious, and hostile
   C. allowing themselves to be exposed to some minor doses of frustration, but are unable to handle the feelings which are produced by the frustration
   D.) A and C (24:90,91)

285. Which of the following signs would appear least indicative of an infant's unpleasant experience with weaning?
   A. seeking contact with surrounding adults
   B. excessive thumbsucking
   C. irritability and crying spells
   D. sleeplessness and playfulness (13:314)

286. Which of the following statements is *not* true concerning suicidal attempts and suicide in children and adolescents?
   A. suicide is more common in males than females
   B. females make more suicidal attempts than males
   C. adolescents who threaten or commit suicide are, in general, impulsive and immature persons
   D.) suicide occurs most often in the age group which ranges from 13 to 22 years (13:738,739)

287. In the grade-school and adolescent groups, depression is often evidenced by
   A. disobedience, continued temper tantrums, accident proneness
   B. aggression, sexual promiscuity, lying
   C. boredom, restlessness, running away from home and school
   D.) A and C (13:739)

288. The basic difference between traumatic and signal anxiety lies in what aspect of the threatening event?

A. source
B.) timing
C. quality
D. quantity (10:339)

Directions: Match the following numbered items with the most appropriate lettered items.

B 289. Embodies a need for recognition and attention (27:97)
C 290. Response to underlying fear of criticism, humiliation, and rejection (27:99)
A 291. Experienced upon failing to meet goals (27:104,105)
C 292. Mechanism used by child who "never causes any trouble" (27:99)
D 293. A preschooler suddenly ceases intelligible speech and reverts to babyish babbling (27:102)

A. Frustration
B. Aggression
C. Isolation
D. Regression

C. Screening Tests

Directions: For each of the following multiple choice questions, select the ONE most appropriate answer.

294. Two screening tests that should be done on all children over 6 months of age are
   A.) cover test and Hirschberg's test
   B. Hirschberg's test and Snellen test
   C. Snellen test and cover test
   D. Ishihara color blindness test and cover test (1:59,60)

295. A constricted pupil may indicate
   A. retinoblastoma
   B. glaucoma
   C. atropine poisoning
   D.) morphine poisoning (1:61)

296. When looking into the distance, the pupils should
   A. constrict
   B.) dilate

C. have no change
D. look irregular (1:62)

297. The permanent color of the iris will be manifested in all children by what age?
A. six months
B. one year
C. eighteen months
D. two years (1:62)

298. The instrument that is necessary for the internal examination of the eyes is the
A. otoscope
B. flashlight
C. ophthalmoscope
D. stethoscope (1:65,66)

299. Observation of the red reflex tells you the child has
A. clear lenses
B. binocular fixation
C. hyperopia
D. increased intracranial pressure (1:64)

300. The Snellen E Chart is generally used to test the vision of
A. adults and children
B. all school age children
C. only those persons who know the alphabet
D. preschoolers, kindergartners and first graders (10:424,428)

301. Home vision tests for children ages one to seven years can be done very well by the use of
A. color blindness test and Snellen E test
B. Snellen E and candy bead tests
C. color blindness and candy bead tests
D. none of the above (5:124)

302. A child reads all the symbols of the Snellen Chart on the 40 foot line. He misses two out of six on the 30 foot line and misses three out of six on the 20 foot line. The acuity is recorded as
A. 20/30
B. 30/20
C. 20/20
D. 20/40 (8:89)

303. Cataracts are the leading cause of blindness in
A. adults
B. children
C. adolescents
D. adults and children (1:62,63)

304. The most important reason for early vision screening is the detection of
A. organic eye disease
B. amblyopia
C. refractive errors
D. B and C (10:425)

305. An eye problem that does not involve a refractive error is
A. astigmatism
B. hyperopia
C. strabismus
D. lateral heterophoria (1:59,60)

306. Manifestations of visual difficulty include the following signs, except
A. frequent or continuous frowning
B. irritability when doing close work
C. inattention during reading periods, chart or map work
D. vomiting just before going to school (5:126)

307. Which of these manifestations is least indicative of visual problems?
A. stumbling over objects
B. frequent complaints of headache
C. tilting head or thrusting head forward when looking at objects
D. frequent rubbing of the eyes (5:126)

308. A Snellen test finding of 20/40 indicates
A. "normal vision"
B. an unusually high degree of visual acuity
C. that the 20 foot line is the smallest line read correctly at a distance of 40 feet
D. that the 40 foot line is the smallest line read correctly at a distance of 20 feet (8:89)

309. Which of the following actions is *not* appropriate for nurses to take?

A. refer all pupils found to have 20/40 or worse vision in one or both eyes
B. do not refer pupils with 20/30 vision who already wear glasses if correction was recently made
C. refer all pupils verified by second screening to have 20/30 or worse in both eyes, or 20/40 or worse in one or both eyes
D. repeat screening should be done on all fourth through sixth grade pupils 20/30 or worse in both eyes, or 20/40 or worse in one or both eyes (8:90)

310. Concerning the Snellen test, if a student wears glasses, he must be screened
A. without glasses first, then with glasses
B. with glasses only
C. without glasses and make note
D. with glasses only upon doctor's order (8:88)

311. Which of the following tests screen children for color blindness?
A. Maddox Rod test
B. Snellen test
C. Ishihara test
D. convex lens test (7:225)

312. Which test below requires reading of test objects on a chart from a measured distance of 20 feet?
A. Maddox Rod test
B. Snellen test
C. Ishihara test
D. convex lens test (5:57)

313. The purposes of a vision-screening program include the following, *except* to
A. discover and insure proper correction of eye defects
B. provide positive learning experiences in eye health for all students
C. make appropriate adjustments in students' school health program
D. train paraprofessional workers for administering screening test (5:56)

314. The Snellen test has several distinct advantages for use in schools. Which one below is not true about the test?

A. it tests both visual acuity and refractive errors
B. it is inexpensive
C. it requires no special electrical apparatus
D. it is easy to administer (5:56,57)

315. Which of the following findings in a hearing test would necessitate referral?
A. loss of more than 20 db in 2 frequencies in one ear
B. loss of less than 30 db in any frequencies
C. loss of more than 20 db in any frequencies
D. A and C (5:72)

316. Which of the following statements is true about visual impairment?
A. between 5 and 10 percent of preschool children have some kind of vision impairment
B. amblyopia affects 10 to 15 percent of children
C. 80 percent of blindness is due to congenital causes
D. vision defects are fortunately rare during childhood (10:425)

317. The cover eye test is primarily to detect
A. amblyopia
B. ptosis
C. heterophia
D. myopia (10:428)

318. In general, referral to an ophthalmologist should be made if vision in either eye is less than
A. 20/50 in preschool children
B. 20/40 in preschool children
C. 20/30 in school-age children
D. 20/60 in adolescents (10:428)

319. Vision testing in children under five years generally
A. involves patience and skill
B. does not give reliable results
C. requires repeat examination to verify suspected defect
D. A and C (10:428)

Health Maintenance and Promotion

320. Which of the following tests is a useful screening device to assess a four- or five-year-old child's readiness for school?
A. Draw-a-man test
B. Ishihara color blindness test
C. Snellen test
D. Stanford-Binet test (10:431)

321. Under six months of age, routine screening for anemia is not indicated except for prematures or children who have had hemolytic disease of the newborn. Which of the following is the average hemoglobin level at five years of age?
A. 10 gm/100 ml
B. 13.5 gm/100 ml
C. 15 gm/100 ml
D. 17.5 gm/100 ml (10:431)

322. In the United States, screening for sickle cell trait or disease is a *must* for which of the groups below?
A. American Indians
B. Asians
C. Negroes
D. Latin Americans (10:432)

323. Screening for phenylketonuria is done by a
A. complete urinalysis
B. complete blood test
C. urine culture
D. capillary blood test (10:433)

324. Screening for lead poisoning is recommended for
A. all children between 18 months and 5 years of age living in old or dilapidated houses
B. children with unexplained vomiting or irritability
C. children with unexplained convulsive seizure
D. all of the above (10:433)

325. Which of the following statements is *not* true about lead poisoning?
A. it is preventable at an early stage
B. once it has reached its clinical stage, the condition is irreversible
C. one-third of children will die once encephalopathy develops

D. two-thirds of survivors will have neurologic sequelae, often severe (10:433)

326. Lead poisoning occurs mostly
A. between 1 and 3 years of age
B. among school-age children
C. between 6 and 12 months of age
D. among preschoolers (10:433)

327. The single most reliable test for lead poisoning is the whole blood lead level. The greatest drawback for use of this is the fact that it
A. is relatively expensive
B. is traumatic to child
C. requires venipuncture
D. requires a few days for completion of test (10:434)

328. Routine tuberculin testing should be done annually in the
A. first 10 years of life
B. first 5 years of life
C. school years through adolescence
D. none of the above (10:434)

329. When should the result of a tuberculin test be read following the inoculation?
A. by the second day
B. by the third day
C. by the fourth day
D. by the fifth day (10:434)

330. Children with learning disabilities share the following characteristics, except
A. average or above average intellectual function
B. adequate sensory acuity
C. low academic achievement
D. impaired sensory acuity (7:469)

331. Mental retardation is best defined as
A. low intelligence quotient of 70 with or without impairment of adaptive behavior
B. sub-average general intellectual functioning associated with impairment in adaptive behavior
C. intelligence quotient below 50 associated with adaptive impairment

D. sub-average specific intellectual functioning associated with anti-social behavior (7:464)

332. Which of the following groups of mental retardates are educable?
A. I.Q. score approximately 40 to 49
B. I.Q. score approximately 30 to 39
(C.) I.Q. score approximately 50 to 70
D. I.Q. score approximately 71 to 80
(7:465)

333. Which of the following groups of mental retardates require custodial care?
A. I.Q. score approximately 40 to 49
B. I.Q. score approximately 30 to 39
(C.) I.Q. score below 30
D. B and C (7:465)

334. Mental retardation is *most* commonly associated with
A. conditions caused by infection
B. diseases caused by intoxication
C. conditions caused by physical agents
(D.) psychologic cause with functional or behavioral reactions (7:465)

335. Which of the following tests is commonly used to classify mental retardation according to symptom severity?
(A.) Stanford-Binet test
B. Denver Developmental Screening test
C. Illinois Test of Psycholinguistic Abilities
D. Gesell Developmental Schedules
(7:466)

336. Socialization and independence are gained by mentally retarded children in the school setting
A. through experiences especially designed for them
(B.) through experiences similar to those of all other children
C. by placing them in regular classes with all other children
D. by involving them in regular school programs (7:466)

337. Children with Stanford-Binet scores below 20 are classified as

(A.) profoundly mentally retarded
B. severely mentally retarded
C. moderately mentally retarded
D. none of the above (7:466)

338. Based on a normally distributed statistical curve, the largest proportion of mentally retarded children are in which group?
(A.) mildly mentally retarded
B. borderline mentally retarded
C. moderately mentally retarded
D. severely mentally retarded (7:466)

339. Which of the following activities is *not* appropriate for the trainable mentally retarded child?
A. setting table for family meals
B. receiving payment for services rendered
C. obtaining ordered items from kitchen
(D.) none of the above (7:467)

340. Acoustically handicapped pupils include the hard-of-hearing and the deaf. The deaf are those with hearing losses of
(A.) more than 70 decibels
B. 50 to 70 decibels
C. 70 decibels with some residual hearing ability
D. B and C (29:134)

341. Ideally, how often should the hearing of all pupils be checked by means of a screening test?
A. every six months
(B.) every year
C. every two years
D. every three years (29:105)

342. Which of the following factors should be essentially considered in formulating a screening test program?
A. facilities
B. tester and pupils to be tested
C. recording of results and follow-up procedures
(D.) all of the above (29:105)

343. The major aim in the education of the deaf is to
(A.) establish a means of communication

B. develop self-sufficiency
C. enhance intellectual power
D. promote interpersonal relations (7:473)

344. Which of the following is not a measure to prevent hearing loss in children?
A. avoidance of swimming by child with perforation of the eardrum
B. appropriate management of acute upper respiratory infection
C. prompt and adequate treatment of otitis media
D. continuous exposure to loud noise (7:472,473)

345. When administering ear drops to an infant, it is necessary to pull his ear
A. up and back
B. down and back
C. straight up
D. straight down (13:330)

346. Which of the following symptoms would be least indicative of otitis media, right ear?
A. bulging tympanic membrane
B. crying when right ear is touched
C. temperature of 104° F
D. bony landmarks obliterated (13:330)

347. Which of the following is *least* likely to cause hearing loss during childhood?
A. accidental injury
B. noise damage
C. foreign bodies in ear canal
D. nutritional deficiency (7:473)

348. Nerve deafness differs from conduction deafness in that the former
A. affects only the elderly
B. can be caused by a general aging process
C. results from blocked eustachian tubes
D. is caused by damage to the ossicles and cochlea (7:472)

349. A child who has an *extreme* hearing loss may
A. misunderstand most of a conversation
B. hear voices only when source is a few inches from his ear
C. hear a shout one inch away from his ear
D. need special assistance in voice development (7:473)

350. A severe hearing loss reflects a hearing level of
A. 41–55 db
B. 56–70 db
C. 71–90 db
D. 91 db or more (7:472)

351. A person beginning to respond to audiometric testing at 15 decibels
A. has slight hearing impairment
B. has no hearing impairment
C. is almost deaf
D. is severely deaf (7:472)

352. If a child does not respond to audiometric testing within normal limits of hearing, he should be
A. referred to an otologist
B. retested another time and day
C. retested by another person
D. retested by another machine (5:67)

353. When examining the tympanic membrane, the nurse is looking for the following characteristics, except
A. color
B. light reflex
C. long and short process
D. texture (1:79)

354. The color of the tympanic membrane is normally
A. light, pearly gray, translucent
B. orange-red uniformly distributed
C. light orange, red or gray background
D. light, dull gray (1:79)

355. The examiner should always test for mobility of the eardrum. A normal tympanic membrane covering only air in the middle ear will
A. not move if pressure is applied
B. move in a shaky or jerky fashion
C. move if slight pressure is applied
D. not move at all (1:79)

356. Which type of hearing loss involves a lesion in the external ear, the middle ear or both?
    A. sensorineural
    B. conductive
    C. pressure
    D. mixed (10:554)

357. The most common cause of conductive impairment is
    A. congenital anomaly
    B. infection
    C. accumulation of cerumen
    D. trauma (29:94)

358. The portion of the ear protruding from the head is called the
    A. annulus
    B. pinna
    C. concha
    D. helix (1:84)

359. Which cranial bone contains the middle ear?
    A. temporal
    B. frontal
    C. parietal
    D. occipital (1:85)

360. The innermost of the three ossicle bones resembling a stirrup is called the
    A. malleus
    B. incus
    C. stapes
    D. umbo (1:74)

361. The main parts of the inner ear are the following, except the
    A. vestibule
    B. semicircular canals
    C. cochlea
    D. tympanic membrane (1:73)

362. What is the technique used for examining the ear of an older child for *best* view of the ear canal?
    A. firmly grip the pinna and pull the ear down
    B. firmly grasp the pinna and pull the ear back
    C. firmly grip the pinna and pull the ear up and back
    D. firmly grasp the pinna and pull the ear down and front (1:76)

363. What structure connects the middle ear with the nasal cavity?
    A. eustachian tube
    B. external meatus
    C. semicircular canals
    D. cochlea (29:94)

364. Which of the following is least likely to cause otitis media?
    A. upper respiratory infection, such as measles, mumps or a common cold
    B. pinching nostrils while blowing or blowing too forcibly
    C. improper functioning of the eustachian tube
    D. lobar pneumonia (29:95,96)

365. Unchecked otitis media can readily produce a very dangerous complication which is
    A. mastoiditis
    B. encephalitis
    C. septicemia
    D. migratory arthritis (29:95,96)

366. A disease that causes a progressive loss of hearing in those afflicted is called
    A. osteoporosis
    B. otosclerosis
    C. otitis media
    D. mastoiditis (29:97)

367. An operative procedure developed to overcome the conductive blockage caused by the aforenoted condition is
    A. mastoidectomy
    B. laminectomy
    C. stapedectomy
    D. stapedotomy (29:97)

368. Which of the following structures represents the end organ for hearing?
    A. vestibular mechanism
    B. incus
    C. maleus
    D. cochlea (29:97)

Health Maintenance and Promotion

369. Which of the following is *least* likely to cause profound hearing impairment?
    A. exposure to sudden loud noise
    B. meningitis and vascular disturbances
    C. measles and mumps
    D. malnutrition (29:97)

370. Which of the following is true about sensorineural hearing impairment?
    A. it is not amenable to medical or surgical care
    B. its acuity for high pitches is frequently *more* than acuity for middle or low pitches
    C. pressure on the nerve of hearing from a brain tumor will cause a sensorineural loss, usually in both ears
    D. it is a common type of hearing problem found in school-age children (29:98)

371. Measurements of hearing acuity are best made with a (an)
    A. otoscope
    B. tuning fork
    C. audiometer
    D. ophthalmoscope (29:99)

372. A child should be suspected of a hearing problem if he presents one or more of the following conditions, except
    A. failure to respond to conversation when head is turned away
    B. frequent requests for repetition of word or sound
    C. faulty pronunciation of rarely used words
    D. unusual dependence on visual cues (29:98)

373. Which of the following is a positive sign of ear, nose and throat difficulties?
    A. persistent mouth breathing
    B. unexplained decrease in school achievement
    C. inattention, restlessness, aggressiveness or apathy
    D. failure to follow directions (29:98)

374. In an audiometric test, which of the following at each frequency represents the intensity required for the average normal ear to detect the presence of a tone?
    A. −10 db
    B. +10 db
    C. zero db
    D. +5 db (29:99)

375. If a child consistently fails to hear 500 cps at the screening level employed, while responding without difficulty to higher frequencies, it is likely that which one of the following factors is present?
    A. room or outside noise is interfering with the accuracy
    B. examiner's technique is faulty
    C. calibration of the audiometer is inaccurate
    D. child is not concentrating on the procedure (29:100)

376. Pupils who fail to respond to one or more frequencies in either ear in the screening test should be given a
    A. perceptual test
    B. complete medical examination of the ear
    C. repeat test
    D. threshold test (29:100)

377. Which of the following frequencies on the audiogram have been found to have a high correlation between the average hearing level at these frequencies and an individual's ability to hear speech?
    A. 500, 1500, 2500 cps
    B. 500, 1000, 2000 cps
    C. 1000, 2000, 3000 cps
    D. 1000, 1500, 2000 cps (7:472)

378. The purpose of the threshold test performed in a school hearing test program is to
    A. determine whether or not a child who failed the screening test needs medical examination of the ears
    B. comply with school health policies
    C. check reliability of the screening test
    D. identify individuals whose hearing at one or more frequencies is outside the range of normal (29:103)

379. The first responsibility of the school nurse when a child has been identified with a hearing impairment is to
    A. refer the child to an otologist for further work-up
    B. arrange for a diagnostic evaluation and any necessary treatment through community resources
    C. notify pupil's parents of his hearing deficit and suggest that he needs a diagnostic examination
    D. forward a report of the school testing results to the family physician
    (29:107)

380. Which of the following agencies certifies the clinical competence of individuals who provide professional services for speech and hearing handicaps?
    A. American Speech and Hearing Association
    B. American Academy of Ophthalmology and Otolaryngology
    C. Volta Bureau
    D. American Hearing Society (29:109)

381. Ideally, a child's dental status should be appraised periodically beginning
    A. just before he starts school
    B. as soon as he is sent to first grade
    C. shortly after completion of his deciduous teeth, usually between two and three years of age
    D. following completion of his deciduous teeth, usually between four and five years of age (10:417)

382. Deciduous dentition is usually completed by the end of the toddler period with the child having
    A. twenty deciduous teeth
    B. thirty-two temporary teeth
    C. his first molars
    D. his primary teeth (8:85)

383. The loss of deciduous molars usually occurs at what age?
    A. 10 to 12 years
    B. 7 to 9 years
    C. 4 to 6 years
    D. 13 to 15 years (8:85)

384. Which of the following is least expected in dental development from birth to six months?
    A. lower deciduous incisor eruptions
    B. neonatal teeth
    C. upper deciduous incisor eruptions
    D. Epstein's pearls (8:85)

385. At about what age do the permanent second molars usually erupt?
    A. 14 years
    B. 12 years
    C. 10 years
    D. 8 years (1:102)

386. How many teeth are there in a complete set of permanent dentition?
    A. twenty-eight
    B. thirty
    C. thirty-two
    D. thirty-four (8:85)

387. Girls have more carious lesions than boys of the same age, the difference being attributed to
    A. greater tendency for girls to eat sweets
    B. earlier eruption of teeth in girls than in boys
    C. constitutional predilection
    D. greater tendency for boys to submit to periodic dental check-ups (29:150)

388. Which of the following statements is *not* true about the incidence and prevalence of dental caries in children and youths of the United States?
    A. approximately 30% of 2-year-old children have one or more carious teeth
    B. by the time children reach school age, they have an average of three carious teeth
    C. by the age of sixteen the average youth has seven teeth decayed, missing or filled
    D. the average number of carious teeth increases with age (29:150)

389. Which of the following measures offers the greatest hope for preventing dental caries?
    A. water fluoridation
    B. topical fluoride application

C. tooth brushing
D. reduction of sugar consumption
(29:150)

390. The ultimate decision regarding the education and care of the handicapped child must be made by the
A. doctor
B. nurse
C. child
D. family (7:474)

391. Which of the following considerations should be the central basis for the decision concerning the education of the child with learning handicaps?
A. child's own needs
B. preference of school
C. availability of special education experts
D. preference of family (7:475)

392. The first step in educational diagnosis is determining
A. availability of school facilities
B. extent of child's learning problem
C. exact nature of learning problem
D. nature of environmental factors
(7:469)

D. Immunizations

Directions: For each of the following multiple choice questions, select the ONE most appropriate answer.

393. Which of the following is a true statement regarding immunity and immunizations?
A. routine smallpox vaccination is recommended for individuals in urban areas of the United States
B. active immunity is acquired by newborns due to placental transfer in utero
C. immunization should be given even after the child has had the disease
D. the D.P.T. is immunization for diphtheria, pertussis, and tetanus (13:319)

394. Booster doses of D.P.T. should be given at
A. 12 months and at 6 years
B. 18 months and at 4 to 6 years

C. 18 months and at 2 to 4 years
D. 2 years and 4 to 6 years (13:320)

395. What diseases does the triple antigen vaccine immunize against?
A. measles, mumps and rubella
B. diphtheria, typhoid and pertussis
C. diphtheria, tetanus and pertussis
D. diphtheria, tetanus and polio
(13:319)

396. Which of the following vaccines can be given orally?
A. Salk polio vaccine
B. all vaccines
C. all but the tetanus toxoid
D. Sabin polio vaccine and the D.P.T.
(13:319)

397. German measles vaccine is recommended for all children between ages
A. 1 year and 12 years
B. 4 years and 12 years
C. 3 years and 14 years
D. 2 years and 14 years (13:321)

398. Mumps vaccine is recommended for administration to the following, *except*
A. young boys approaching puberty
B. adult males who have not had mumps
C. children between ages one and twelve years
D. none of the above (13:321)

399. Vaccination against measles is delayed until one year of age because
A. infants are extremely susceptible to any form of viral infection
B. during the first year antibodies transmitted via placental circulation are still present in infants
C. infants are given other kinds of immunizations during first year which may weaken effect of measles immunization
D. febrile period following measles vaccination could endanger life of infant
(13:321)

400. The frequency of repeated tuberculin tests depends on
A. risk of exposure to individual child

B. prevalence of tuberculosis in population group
C. parental consent
D. A and B (13:321)

401. Booster doses of adult type diphtheria-tetanus toxoids should be given at
A. 14 to 16 years, every 10 years thereafter
B. 6 to 12 years, every 10 years thereafter
C. 14 to 18 years, every 5 years thereafter
D. 7 to 14 years, every 5 years thereafter (13:320)

402. If the child is immunized against tetanus, and receives an injury with a dirty wound,
A. an extra dose of tetanus antitoxin should not be given unless he manifests indicative signs of tetanus
B. apply wet dressing to dirty wound; extra dose of tetanus antitoxin is not necessary
C. an extra dose of tetanus antitoxin should be given to provide immediate increase in immunity
D. an extra dose of tetanus antitoxin may be given only with parental consent (11:163)

403. Starting at 6 to 10 weeks of life, all infants should receive which of the following immunizations?
A. diphtheria-pertussis-tetanus combined immunization
B. smallpox vaccine
C. measles vaccine
D. diphtheria-tetanus toxoid (10:435)

404. The main reason for starting the immunization program before the sixth month of life is that newborns do not receive passive immunity against
A. diphtheria
B. tetanus
C. pertussis
D. tetanus and pertussis (10:435)

405. How many months is the time-honored interval between the first three D.P.T. immunizations?
A. 1
B. 1½
C. 2
D. 2½ (10:436)

406. Which of the D.P.T. immunizations is in the form of a vaccine?
A. diphtheria
B. pertussis
C. tetanus
D. none of the above (10:436)

407. What is the sensitivity test for diphtheria?
A. Schick
B. Dick
C. Tine
D. BCG (10:436)

408. The preferred site for smallpox vaccination is the skin near the insertion of the
A. gluteus maximus
B. biceps
C. deltoid
D. triceps (10:437)

409. With infants still in diapers, the thigh should be avoided for smallpox vaccination because of
A. extreme pain in this area
B. underdeveloped muscles
C. danger of secondary bacterial infection
D. danger of hitting sciatic nerve (10:437)

410. Under what conditions should there be *no* contraindication to smallpox vaccination?
A. by end of first year of life
B. presence of epidemic or known exposure
C. travel abroad and within three years of reentry into the United States
D. B and C (11:163)

411. Gamma globulin affords
A. permanent protection against certain virus infection
B. temporary protection against poliomyelitis
C. immediate overall protection against bacterial and viral infections
D. temporary protection against certain virus infection (11:164)

Health Maintenance and Promotion

412. No reaction to smallpox vaccination indicates an unsuccessful vaccination which may be due to
    A. faulty technique
    B. dead vaccine
    C. none of the above
    D. A and B   (10:437)

413. A primary reaction, which indicates lack of previous immunity, reaches a peak of how many days?
    A. 8 to 12
    B. 5 to 10
    C. 14 to 18
    D. 16 to 21   (10:437)

414. The reaction site in smallpox vaccination should be observed how many weeks after immunization?
    A. one
    B. two
    C. three
    D. four   (10:437)

415. To what age group is measles vaccine usually administered in the United States?
    A. one year to eighteen months
    B. nine months to one year
    C. six months to eight months
    D. eighteen months to two years (10:438)

416. Which of the following tests should be administered before measles vaccination?
    A. Schick test
    B. Maloney test
    C. Schwartz test
    D. tuberculin test   (10:438)

417. Which of the following statements is *not* true about measles vaccination?
    A. live measles vaccine should not be administered to a pregnant woman if the patient has received gamma globulin within six weeks
    B. live measles vaccine should not be administered during pregnancy if there is marked egg sensitivity
    C. children with altered immune responses should be administered with live *but* highly attenuated vaccines
    D. measles is now preventable, and all infants and susceptible children should receive one of the live, attenuated vaccines available (10:438)

418. Which of the following immunizing agents are recommended for routine use in *all* children in the United States?
    A. D.P.T., trivalent O.P.V., measles, D.P.T. booster
    B. measles, D.P.T., trivalent O.P.V., B.C.G.
    C. D.T. booster, smallpox, influenza
    D. A and C   (10:438)

419. Which of the following is an accurate statement about poliomyelitis immunization?
    A. the safety and effectiveness of live attenuated poliomyelitis vaccine has not been established
    B. at least three administrations are recommended during the first eighteen months of life, which will result in nearly 100 percent immunity
    C. pregnant women and young adults should *not* receive a full immunization course
    D. the immunization is administered by parenteral route (10:437,438)

420. Which of the following statements should be emphasized in explaining immunization to a mother?
    A. in smallpox vaccination of young babies, complications seem to occur less often than in older children vaccinated for the first time
    B. when a child is given tetanus toxoid in infancy and gets the proper booster, he may not need tetanus antitoxin later if he receives an injury, but he will need toxoid and will be more effectively protected
    C. explain the schedule of future inoculations
    D. all of the above   (11:76,77)

421. Which of the following approaches is likely to be *least* effective in making immunization procedures less unpleasant for the child?

A. let child watch injection if he wants to
B. be sure needle is sharp
C. do not stretch or hold skin before inserting needle
D. inject older child last (11:76)

422. The best sites for administering the D.P.T. vaccine are
A. lower, outer side of thigh or arm
B. upper, outer side of thigh or arm
C. upper, outer quadrant of buttocks
D. none of the above (11:162)

423. A very important consideration to observe after administering D.P.T. immunization is to
A. apply gauze patch over the site
B. avoid massage of the site
C. press sponge on skin over needle
D. B and C (11:162)

424. Which of the following agents provides a passive immunization to the recipient?
A. D.P.T. vaccine
B. trivalent O.P.V. vaccine
C. gamma globulin
D. smallpox vaccine (11:164)

425. Which of the following immunizing agents is *not* routinely used in the United States, but is usually required for travel overseas or for continuous exposure to unsanitary environment?
A. dysentery vaccine
B. typhoid fever vaccine
C. typhus vaccine
D. yellow fever vaccine (11:164)

426. Communicable diseases which are usually mild during childhood but are especially hazardous to certain adults are
A. varicella and influenza
B. mumps and rubella
C. poliomyelitis and encephalitis
D. tetanus and meningitis (11:164)

427. Which of the following points should generally be included in anticipatory counseling regarding a child's inoculation?
A. only a few children show a real reaction with pain and fever to the inoculation and any such reaction will develop in 6 to 24 hours after the inoculation
B. any illness occurring later than this 6 to 24 hour period is apt to be a real illness
C. fever and general sick feeling can be eased by small doses of aspirin; if it is not relieved, consult doctor
D. all of the above (11:167)

428. A successful smallpox vaccination should show one of the following reactions, except
A. "primary take"
B. "no-take"
C. "immune reaction"
D. "accelerated reaction" (11:167)

429. Which of the following reactions would indicate that the smallpox vaccination acted as a booster?
A. "immune reaction"
B. "accelerated reaction"
C. "primary take"
D. "no-take" (11:167)

430. Which of the following is contraindicated in the care of smallpox vaccination?
A. bathe child daily but with shower or sponge bath
B. vaccination site may get wet but it should not be allowed to soak in bath water
C. wear a long-sleeved shirt to prevent scratching
D. apply soothing ointment if vaccinated area gets itchy (11:167)

Directions: This part of the test consists of a situation followed by a series of incomplete statements. Study the situation and select the best answer to complete each statement that follows.

Situation: You are working with a mother of a newborn and are planning an immunization program with her. She asks the following questions:

431. I've heard the terms "active" and "passive" immunization. I don't understand the difference. Can you tell me?
A. in "active" immunity, the person develops his own defense (antibodies)

against the causative organism (antigen)
B. in "passive" immunity, the person must receive the defense (antibodies) from someone else
C. serums contain the defense (antibodies) and give "passive" immunity
D. all of the above (11:161,164)

432. By the end of the first year, which immunizations should my baby receive?
A. triple antigen vaccine
B. trivalent oral polio virus vaccine
C. measles-rubella vaccine
D. all of the above (10:438)

433. Which diseases does the triple antigen vaccine immunize against?
A. measles, mumps and rubella
B. diphtheria, typhoid and pertussis
C. diphtheria, tetanus and pertussis
D. diphtheria, tetanus and polio (10:438)

434. Can any of the vaccines be given orally?
A. yes, the trivalent oral polio vaccine
B. yes, all of them
C. yes, all but the tetanus toxoid
D. yes, the trivalent oral polio vaccine and the D.T.P. (10:438)

435. When will my child need a booster shot of tetanus after she has received her initial three injections?
A. if more than 10 years have elapsed since the last dose in a clean minor wound
B. if more than 5 years have elapsed since the last dose in a contaminated wound
C. never, since the initial series provides permanent immunization
D. A and B (13:319)

E. Nutrition

Directions: For each of the following multiple choice questions, select the ONE most appropriate answer.

436. Approximately how many calories per day is required for a 6-month-old baby?
A. 50 cal/lb
B. 70 cal/lb
C. 80 cal/lb
D. 100 cal/lb (28:34)

437. The most essential element in the diet of children and adolescents is
A. proteins
B. carbohydrates
C. water
D. vitamins (28:34)

438. Which of the following elements are required for the production of antibodies and for cellular structure?
A. minerals
B. proteins
C. carbohydrates
D. vitamins (28:35)

439. Which of the following statements is true about carbohydrates, when comparing breast milk with cow's milk?
A. carbohydrate content is greater in breast milk
B. carbohydrate content is less in breast milk
C. each type has equal amounts of carbohydrates
D. each type has different kinds of carbohydrates (28:36)

440. Both cow's milk and breast milk have the
A. same caloric value per ounce and same amount of fat
B. same amount of fat and vitamin content
C. same kind of carbohydrate and mineral content
D. none of the above (28:36)

441. Which of the following statements is true about digestion of human milk as compared with cow's milk?
A. it is the same for both human and cow's milk
B. it is more rapid in human milk than in cow's milk
C. it is more rapid in cow's milk than in human milk
D. it is undetermined (28:36)

442. Liver, raisins and prunes are a rich source of
A. vitamin A

B. vitamin C
C. calcium
D. iron ✓ (28:35)

443. Which of the following food groups yield the highest protein content?
A. eggs, carrots, dried fruits, spinach
B. poultry, fish, beef, peanut butter ✓
C. beef, broccoli, carrots, dried fruits
D. milk, bread, fish, spinach (28:34)

444. Spaghetti, bread, and danish rolls offer a rich supply of
A. carbohydrates ✓
B. proteins
C. minerals
D. vitamins (8:67)

445. The outstanding disadvantages of most commercial formula preparations are that they
a. need refrigeration
b. are costly
c. require good technique in preparation
d. contain demineralized whey proteins
    A. a and b
    B. b and c
    C. c and d
    D. b and d ✓ (13:147)

446. Concerning cow's milk, which of the following statements is true?
A. it contains more protein than breast milk ✓
B. it contains less protein than breast milk
C. it contains the same amount of protein as does breast milk
D. it contains a more casein type of protein than breast milk (28:36)

447. Which of the following foods would *not* be restricted on a low phenylalanine diet?
A. hard candy, milk, meat
B. natural fruit juices, wheat cereals, eggs
C. tapioca, margarine, applesauce ✓
D. sugar, fish, natural fruits (13:396)

448. Mrs. K. says that Alex, who has celiac disease, loves "pop tarts" for breakfast. Can he have these? Your best response would be

A. "Let's look at the label and see what they are made of." ✓
B. "Since this is not a cereal, you can go ahead and give them to him."
C. "Let Alex try them and watch his stools to see how he reacts."
D. "*Pop tarts* are mostly empty calories so you need not be concerned." (13:373)

449. What is the best approach for introducing new foods to a school-age child?
A. provide a choice
B. make serving as attractive as possible ✓
C. introduce it in a group of peers
D. express understanding about the child's resistance (13:625–26)

450. During the adolescent period, approximately how much of the total daily caloric intake should be derived from protein?
A. 40%
B. 30%
C. 20%
D. 15% ✓ (13:695)

451. Because of rapid growth, the adolescent girl may need 2400 calories daily and the boy
A. 2000 calories
B. 2400 calories
C. 3000 calories ✓
D. 3400 calories (13:694)

452. The adolescent should receive up to 60 gm. of protein a day, the best sources being
A. milk, eggs, meat and cheese ✓
B. tapioca, butter, vegetables, and cheese
C. cream, fruits, meat, and fish
D. bread, meat, fish, and eggs (13:694)

453. Which of the statements below is true about the eating practices of school children?
A. their eating problems relate mostly to content and amount of food consumed
B. they usually eat well and have fewer food fads than preschool children ✓
C. seven-year-old children tend to talk much during meals
D. ten- to twelve-year-old children are apt to have better table manners in public than at home (13:626)

Directions: Match the following numbered items with the most appropriate lettered items.

454. Essential for maintaining acid-base balance (28:34)
455. Utilized for bone formation and enzyme production (28:35)
456. For regulation of body temperature (28:34)
457. Best source of energy for work and play (28:34)
458. Related to hardness of bones and teeth (28:35)
459. Essential for new tissue formation (28:34)
460. Necessary for production of gastric hydrochloric acid (28:35)

    A. Proteins
    B. Carbohydrates
    C. Water
    D. Minerals

Directions: For each of the following multiple choice questions, select the ONE most appropriate answer.

461. Which of the following foods offer the most calcium content?
    A. carrots, milk, eggs, fish
    B. clams, green leafy vegetables, cheese, spaghetti
    C. milk, leafy vegetables, clams, fish
    D. whole grains, raisins, nuts, egg yolk (28:35)

462. Vitamin C deficiency may be manifested by
    A. gingival edema, rachitic rosary, anorexia
    B. ecchymoses, gingival tenderness, bleeding from mucous membranes
    C. subperiosteal hemorrhages, hot-cross-bun skull, pigeon breast
    D. irritability, abdominal distention, cheilosis (28:54,55)

463. During the school age, caloric requirements per unit of body weight
    A. continue to decrease, but nutritional requirements remain relatively greater than in the adult
    B. continue to increase but nutritional requirements remain relatively less than in the adult
    C. continue to decrease and nutritional requirements remain relatively the same as in the adult
    D. continue to increase and nutritional requirements remain relatively the same as in the adult (13:625)

464. Which of the following statements does not relate to food appetite?
    A. appetite is necessarily associated with physiologic hunger
    B. appetite is a conditioned response
    C. mere thought of pleasurable food may stimulate appetite by increasing gastric peristalsis and secretions
    D. each child experiences normal periods of reduced physiologic hunger associated with periods of appetite wanings (27:1)

465. The guidelines below are helpful in minimizing feeding problems, *except that*
    A. child should be prepared for food by pleasant anticipatory conversation and the food presented without undue delay
    B. all toys and any unappetizing odors or sights should be removed and the stage set for eating as the activity of the moment
    C. servings should be a little more than that which could be consumed by the child and left-over food removed without further comment
    D. toddlers and older children should be allowed to leave the table when they have finished eating (27:3)

466. Which of the following sequences is most advisable when adding new foods to the infant's diet?
    A. cereal, vegetables, egg yolks
    B. vegetables, meat, whole eggs
    C. fruit, meat, fish
    D. cereal, fruit, meat (27:4)

467. The following signs are highly suggestive of a child's intolerance to a particular food, *except*

A. fever or drowsiness
B. excessive flatus or excessive stooling
C. regurgitating or vomiting
D. rash or irritability (27:4)

468. Which of the following foods should be omitted from the child's diet until his digestive system has developed sufficiently to accommodate them?
A. peach, pear, milk, orange juice
B. beef with noodles, lamb with peas, macaroni with egg yolk
C. sweet potatoes, squash, onions, pepper
D. spinach, beans, chicken and noodles, turkey and noodles (27:4)

469. Which one of the statements below is *not pertinent* to the management of adolescent obesity?
A. know content of adolescent's present diet as accurately as possible before giving out nutritional counseling
B. convert his diet history into calories by assigning foods to basic four food groups
C. correlate his physical measurements with standard height and weight chart
D. give him a dietary regimen and require him to follow it until further advice (8:61)

470. To lose one pound a week, an individual needs to decrease his daily intake by
A. 400 calories
B. 500 calories
C. 600 calories
D. 700 calories (8:61)

471. The maximum weight loss per week for any individual on diet should not exceed
A. 5 pounds
B. 4 pounds
C. 3 pounds
D. 2 pounds (8:61)

472. Obesity is rarely an isolated problem. Which factor below is least associated with the excessive weight condition?
A. need for attention
B. use of food as behavioral reward
C. unexpected vacation
D. overprotection from mother (8:62)

Directions: Match the following numbered items with the most appropriate lettered items.

473. Egg (8:65)
474. Milk (8:65)
475. Spaghetti (8:67)
476. Carrots (8:65)
477. Poultry (8:65)
478. Spinach (8:66)
479. Fish (8:65)
480. Bread (8:67)
481. Dried fruits (8:66)
482. Peanut butter (8:65)

A. Carbohydrates
B. Proteins
C. Minerals
D. Vitamins

483. Strawberries (8:66)
484. Broccoli (8:66)
485. Ice cream (8:65)
486. Liver (8:66)
487. Raisins (8:66)
488. Spinach (8:66)
489. Cottage cheese (8:65)
490. Tomatoes (8:66)
491. Cantaloupe (8:66)
492. Prunes (8:66)

A. Vitamin A
B. Vitamin C
C. Calcium
D. Iron

Directions: For each of the following multiple choice questions, select the ONE most appropriate answer.

493. Which of the following is least associated with poor appetites in children?
A. overprotective parents
B. lack of food choices
C. timing of snacks
D. growth spurts (27:2)

494. Colic may be caused by one or a combination of the following factors, *except*
A. excessive intake of carbohydrates
B. excessive air swallowing
C. underfeeding
D. emotional tension in infant (13:313)

Health Maintenance and Promotion 87

495. At the end of the first year, the child's appetite will decrease primarily because of his
    A. increasing activity
    B. slower rate of growth
    C. developing other skills
    D. increasing interest in play   (13:313)

496. At five to six months, the average infant
    A. begins to use his fingers in eating
    B. has acquired the skill of holding a spoon and playing with it
    C. holds his own bottle and seems to prefer doing so
    D. wants his bottle at bedtime for comfort of sucking   (13:313)

497. The best time for weaning is generally in the
    A. first half of the second year
    B. second third of the second year
    C. second half of the first year
    D. second third of the first year   (13:314)

498. Under what condition should weaning *never* be undertaken?
    A. when mother is chronically ill
    B. when mother is pregnant
    C. when sibling is hospitalized for tonsillectomy
    D. when infant is sick or hospitalized   (13:314)

499. Which of the following factors is *least* likely to explain a preschooler's refusal to eat sufficient food at mealtimes?
    A. limited snacks
    B. overfatigue
    C. emotional disturbance
    D. imitation of adults who have poor appetites   (13:542)

500. Which of the following guidelines is *least* helpful in establishing healthy eating habits among preschoolers?
    A. foods which can be picked up in fingers should not be served at regular meals
    B. father should be appreciative of food served
    C. children should not be coaxed, bribed or forced to eat
    D. table conversation should consider child and adult interests   (13:542)

501. Measures which have proved helpful in increasing a child's appetite include
    A. serving meal in quiet environment
    B. providing rest period before meals
    C. using pretty dishes, giving small servings
    D. all of the above   (13:542)

502. Vitamin D is added to the diet when the infant is about two weeks old. In general, what is the daily requirement for vitamin D?
    A. 300 I.U.
    B. 400 I.U.
    C. 500 I.U.
    D. 600 I.U.   (13:310)

503. Anorexia is characterized by
    A. fussiness about food, refusal to eat
    B. irregular mealtime
    C. indiscriminate eating between meals
    D. all of the above   (28:76)

504. Psychologic anorexia may be influenced by the following factors, *except*
    A. oversolicitude regarding child's food
    B. failure to permit and encourage normal feeding pattern
    C. anemia or chronic infection
    D. attention-getting maneuver   (28:76)

505. Which type of vitamin deficiency may be induced by isoniazid therapy?
    A. riboflavin
    B. niacin
    C. biotin
    D. pyridoxine hydrochloride   (28:53)

506. The starvation syndrome occurring when infants consume a diet lacking in sufficient calories is called
    A. marasmus
    B. kwashiorkor
    C. carotenemia
    D. de Toni-Debre Fanconi syndrome   (28:61)

507. The following are signs of kwashiorkor, *except*
    A. diarrhea, edema
    B. irritability, apathy
    C. loose, wrinkled skin — marasmus
    D. sparse, thin hair   (28:61)

508. The richest source of iodine is
    A. meat
    B. seafood
    C. milk
    D. vegetables   (28:35)

509. The most important factor in providing a lunch menu for a group of school-age children is
    A. calories
    B. cultural requirements
    C. fluid requirements
    D. vitamins   (28:44)

F. Health Education and Counseling

Directions: For each of the following multiple choice questions, select the ONE most appropriate answer.

510. Which of the following statements is generally considered a fallacy?
    A. everything the doctor and nurse do is educational
    B. every contact between parents and staff is educational
    C. health education refers to regular parent counseling which takes place as part of conference procedure
    D. health education refers to materials and activities designed to inform parents about health and care of children
                                        (11:136)

511. Group discussions in a conference setting present very real, practical problems which may include the following, *except*
    A. getting mothers together, sharing of experiences
    B. skill of leader, size of group
    C. areas of concern, experimentation with variety of patterns
    D. curriculum development
                                (11:137,138,139)

512. Which of the following materials is *most* effective in implementing a health education unit?
    A. pamphlets and leaflets
    B. exhibits and displays
    C. pictures and posters
    D. films and film strips   (11:139,140,141)

513. Teaching an individual what to expect before she begins to worry or make mistakes is the basic philosophy of
    A. health education
    B. anticipatory guidance
    C. education for child rearing
    D. parent effectiveness training   (11:47)

514. Jealousy of a new baby can be a devastating experience for a child. Which of the following measures is *most likely* to promote sibling jealousy?
    A. make whatever changes necessary *before* new baby comes
    B. have mother bring older child a present upon her return from hospital
    C. plan so that baby is being nursed the first time child sees him
    D. do not always talk about new baby
                                        (11:50)

515. A mother is eager to know whether Kevin, age 6 years, would indeed be a bedwetter all throughout childhood. He has been bedwetting since she came back from the hospital with the new baby. Your best response should be
    A. "Don't worry, he will eventually get over it."
    B. "Ask your pediatrician for specific things to do."
    C. "He feels neglected, that's why he is bedwetting."
    D. "This concerns you, doesn't it? Some return to babyish ways in the older child is not unusual."   (11:50)

516. Because a baby's crying distresses most mothers, it is important to give the mother some facts about crying before it begins to get on her nerves. Which of the following is *hardly* a true statement about crying?
    A. crying is a baby's chief mode of communication

B. every bit of a baby's fussings is an emergency requiring immediate action
C. baby's crying is his signal that he wants something
D. letting a baby cry a few minutes is not the same as letting him cry for hours (11:53)

517. Most babies eat and sleep according to their needs; therefore, it is best to place a baby on a
A. flexible schedule
B. self-demand feeding
C. self-regulation feeding
D. regimented schedule (11:52)

518. An outstanding characteristic of a two-year-old is the frequent appearance of irrational fears, hence it is best to avoid any potentially traumatic experience for the child. Of the situations below, which one would be least likely traumatic for him?
A. elective operative procedures
B. extended separation from mother
C. mother's taking a job
D. placing child in day care center (11:58)

519. The consequences of maternal deprivation have been described in many studies. Separation is most traumatic for the child under the following conditions, *except* when
A. he is suddenly taken over by strangers whether in his own home or away from it
B. his routines are changed
C. he is provided a mother substitute *minimize*
D. he is hurt or restrained (11:58)

520. It is important to allow the child to use each new ability as it appears. When he is at the "putting-in" and "taking-out" stage, which of the following activities would be the most appropriate for him?
A. attach strings or handles to pushable objects
B. find some safe steps so he can go up and down
C. give him lots of pots and pans, blocks, bowls and boxes
D. put empty cup and dish on his tray for him to play with (11:62)

521. A father tells you that he is quite disturbed about his son's behavior lately. He has been saying to him "you stink." Your response should be
A. "Take him to the clinic tomorrow. I'll give him an assessment."
B. "Refer him to your doctor; he can give you specific ways to deal with your child."
C. "Don't you worry. He does not really mean what he's saying."
D. "I understand; however, your child's seeming defiance is an aspect of growth and he will eventually outgrow this. It is best to ignore it." (11:62)

522. Parents frequently worry about the gait, the posture and the feet as the child starts standing and walking. Which of the statements below is true about an infant's posture and gait?
A. infantile bowleg becomes a mild knock knee at about 18 months and persists through 3 years
B. infant's knock knee is marked at one year and persists through 2½ years
C. usually knock knee will correct itself by 7 years
D. flatfoot and toe-in or toe-out during conversion to a biped position should have orthopedic treatment (11:73)

523. Mrs. White just learned that her daughter Janet has chicken pox. The nurse should instruct Mrs. White to
a. keep Janet in bed in her own room and keep other children away
b. not send other children to school until Janet is well
c. boil Janet's dishes after each meal
d. apply an antiseptic lotion to the lesions to prevent scarring
A. all of the above
B. a, b, and c
C. a and c
D. all but d (13:561,568)

524. Mrs. Garver asked the public health nurse at the well-child conference when it would be appropriate to begin to toilet train her one-year-old son. Which of the following

statements should be the best response for the nurse?
A. "You could start now as your child is physiologically ready."
B. "You can start with urinary control at 18 months and after that is attained work on bowel control."
C. "Bowel control should be attained by 2 years through the use of periodic enemas."
D. "Bowel control can be accomplished by 18 months; however, training should not be attempted during family crisis periods." (13:420,421,422)

525. In helping parents with child rearing, it is best to initially
A. give specific information about child care which the parent should follow
B. reassure parents concerning their child rearing practices
C. ask parents for their own ideas and show them how to use their own resources
D. show parents aspects of their child rearing that need change (10:346)

526. Which of the following statements is *not* true?
A. if a disorder is inherited, a chromosome analysis shows abnormality
B. dominant disorders are frequent; recessive disorders are rare
C. in sex-linked recessive pattern of inheritance, the affected persons are principally females
D. the offspring of closely related persons have a higher probability of showing hereditary disorders (10:189,190)

527. A trait *not due* to an autosomal recessive gene is
A. cleft palate
B. bird-headed dwarf
C. phenylketonuria
D. cystic fibrosis (10:193)

528. The increase in congenital defects is *least* explained by which one of the following?
A. relative increase in vital statistics
B. poor diagnostic procedures
C. better care and survival of defective persons until past their reproductive age
D. prevention of natural abortions (10:190)

529. Most congenital malformations are caused by
A. mendelian factors
B. unifactors
C. multifactors
D. recessive genes (13:185)

530. Which statement does *not* reflect the transmission of sex-linked recessive genes?
A. the incidence of a trait is much higher in males than in females
B. transmission is from father to son
C. transmission is from father to daughter
D. daughters are usually carriers (10:191)

531. If a male patient was observed to have two x-chromosomes by the Barr body test he would probably be diagnosed as being
A. mongoloid
B. hypertrichosic
C. apert
D. klinefelter (10:192)

532. Without a physician's order, the pediatric nurse practitioner may do the following, *except*
A. plan and implement an immunization program
B. follow a child's condition in the hospital
C. develop a teaching program for a diabetic child
D. prescribe an antibiotic for a child with otitis media (5:16,17)

533. Health problems seen especially during preadolescence and adolescence include the following, *except*
A. osteosarcoma
B. rheumatic fever
C. slipped femoral epiphysis
D. Ewing's sarcoma or tuberculosis (13:715,723)

534. An adolescent is concerned about his oily, blemished skin. He asks you what causes

this condition. Which of the following factors would you include in your response to him?
A. familial predisposition
B. overactivity
C. diet and erratic sleep patterns
D. all of the above (13:701,702)

535. A mother is eager to have a brown-eyed baby. Her 6-month-old baby's eyes are blue. She asks you if the color can still change. Which of the following is the best response to her question?
A. "No, eye color doesn't change after 4 weeks."
B. "No, eye color change usually occurs by three months."
C. "Yes, eye color change can occur anytime in the first year."
D. "If you and your husband both have brown eyes, they will change." (1:62)

536. A carrier of a recessive gene can have affected children
A. only if he or she marries a carrier
B. if he marries a close relative
C. if one of the siblings is frankly abnormal
D. if he or she marries somebody carrying a dominant trait of some sort (10:183)

537. John asks you why stretching is a good treatment for his scoliosis. Your best response should be
A. "It applies equal pressure on both sides of the vertebra so bone growth proceeds equally."
B. "It separates vertebrae so that they can slip back into normal position."
C. "It reduces pressure on the compressed side of the vertebra and increases pressure on the concave side so that bone growth can proceed."
D. A and B (10:748)

538. Chronic poor positioning is a precursor to bone deformities. Measures to minimize the incidence of bone deformities associated with paralytic disorders include
A. maintaining full range of motion of all major points daily
B. judiciously using foot boards and hip rolls
C. daily stretching of extremities
D. all of the above (10:510,511)

539. Heredity means the transmission of potential traits from the parents to their children. The genes are carried through the
A. chromosomes
B. sex chromatins
C. DNA
D. RNA (13:181,182)

540. The storehouse of genetic information is believed to be the
A. chromosomes
B. Barr body
C. DNA
D. RNA (13:182)

541. Genes at the same locus on a pair of homologous chromosomes are alleles. When both members of a pair of alleles are present, the individual is
A. heterozygous
B. homozygous
C. dominant
D. recessive (13:183)

542. Which of the following is theoretically true about autosomal recessive inheritance in a family of four children?
A. only one parent is carrier
B. one child will be homozygous normal
C. two children will be heterozygous abnormal
D. one child will be heterozygous abnormal (13:183)

543. The organism is most vulnerable to injury during the
A. fetal period
B. time of fertilization
C. embryonic period
D. neonatal period (13:185)

544. Which of the statements below is *not* true about congenital disease?
A. it is acquired while infant is in utero
B. it is subject to preventive medicine
C. it is fixed at time of conception
D. it includes structural anomalies present at birth (13:186)

Chapter III: Answers and Explanations

1. **B.**—Inasmuch as the umbilicus is completely severed from the maternal circulation, then it should be completely pulseless.
2. **A.**—Approximately 70 to 90 out of every 100 newborns should score 7 or above one minute after birth.
3. **B.**—Abduction on the affected side is limited to no more than 45 degrees.
4. **D.**—The posterior fontanel ordinarily closes by 1 to 2 months of life.
5. **B.**—The maternal hormones would not have any effect on the male genitalia.
6. **C.**—Thrush patches are usually caused by poor oral hygiene and they leave a red bleeding spot when they are scraped off. Bottle-fed babies are prone to thrush infections.
7. **C.**—At 1 year of age the birth weight is tripled.
8. **A.**—Infant's body metabolism is more rapid than that of an adult because of the rapid growth and developmental changes taking place during the first year of life. Death is most often due to the effects of dehydration and to acid-base imbalance.
9. **D.**—Whereas about 53% of the body weight of the adult is made up of water, 70 to 83% of the infant's body weight is composed of water. Dehydration in infants is thus more serious than in the adult.
10. **D.**—A one-month-old infant can turn his head to the side when prone and be able to follow a bright object to the midline. Activity diminishes when he regards a human face.
11. **D.**—Smelling is not a standard method of physical examination.
12. **C.**—Percussion is done by placing the middle finger of one hand against the body part to be percussed and then striking this finger with the index or middle finger of the other hand.
13. **B.**—On the other hand, the finger tips seem to be most discriminating in fine tactile details.
14. **A.**—This is probably because we are so used to inspecting in everyday life in a rather haphazard manner.
15. **D.**—In addition, the general atmosphere should be warm, friendly, and unhurried.
16. **D.**—The child should be allowed to adjust gradually to the situation.
17. **B.**—Undressing the child all at once is a very poor technique with preschoolers. This is the age group when children are first aware of sexual modesty and, as such, are particular about removing their underpants.
18. **A.**—This appears to be a useful system since examination of the ears and throat often results in angry, crying protest.
19. **A.**—It often pays to examine the least fearful child first, giving the others a chance to see just what will happen to them and that it will not be traumatic, and meanwhile letting the first patient feel important by being first.
20. **C.**—Silence could be very threatening to an older child especially upon examination. Children generally love to be talked with.
21. **A.**—The posterior roof of the mouth is called the soft palate.
22. **G.**—Thrush is often treated by the application of any anti-fungal agent.

23. **E.**—Glossitis is generally caused by any type of infection, usually secondary to pharyngitis.
24. **D.**—Caries are a very common health problem and should be checked for at every health examination.
25. **I.**—Halitosis may be due to poor hygiene, a local or systemic infection, sinusitis, mouth breathing, or a foreign body in the nose.
26. **C.**—Epstein's pearls are also called Bohn nodules when on the midplate. Both types usually disappear in 2 or 3 months.
27. **B.**—Cheilitis may be due to wind and sun. Children with upper respiratory infections and febrile illness are prone to cheilitis.
28. **L.**—Cold sores may present an inflamed base with burning and itching. Eating is painful.
29. **H.**—Glossoptosis is frequently accompanied by a small mandible resulting in feeding problems, hypoxia, cyanosis and dyspnea.
30. **F.**—If a child has unexplained dysphagia, the base of the tongue should be examined for possible congenital anomaly.
31. **A.**—Blood is supplied to the mouth through the facial, lingual and maxillary branches of the external carotid artery.
32. **D.**—The fifth cranial nerve (trigeminal) and the seventh cranial nerve (facial) are the two main nerves that supply the innervation of the oral cavity.
33. **D.**—The laryngopharynx lies between the oropharynx and the cricoid cartilage and esophagus.
34. **C.**—The parotid gland lies in front of and below the external ear.
35. **B.**—Infants usually drool for several months until they learn how to swallow saliva.
36. **A.**—The crown is composed of enamel.
37. **D.**—The deciduous teeth are otherwise known as temporary or milk teeth.
38. **B.**—The first teeth may not erupt until 12 months.
39. **C.**—Around the end of the sixth year the first molars begin to erupt.
40. **B.**—Bright cherry-red lips may be indicative of acidosis from aspirin poisoning, diabetes or carbon monoxide poisoning.
41. **D.**—Halitosis, associated with a specific illness, usually clears up when the child regains his health and begins to eat and drink normally.
42. **C.**—Some diseases give off distinct breath smell. Just as uremia gives off an ammoniacal smell, typhoid fever smells like decaying tissue.
43. **D.**—Excess iron ingestion usually results in green and black teeth, but this discoloration will disappear as soon as the child's diet contains less iron.
44. **B.**—The white strawberry tongue occurs on the second to third day of scarlet fever, but it sometimes occurs in measles or other febrile diseases.
45. **D.**—Impairment of the twelfth cranial nerve causes displacement of the tongue so that it is very important to examine the status of this nerve if neoplasm has been ruled out.
46. **A.**—Spitting up blood from the lungs is called hemoptysis.
47. **C.**—The maxillary sinuses are located along the lateral wall of the nasal cavity.
48. **B.**—The nostrils are the orifices at the base of the nose.
49. **C.**—Only the nose, nasal passages, and paranasal sinuses are accessible to physical examination.
50. **D.**—The procerus inserts between the eyebrows and runs towards the apex of the nose.
51. **A.**—The frontal sinuses develop at approximately 7 to 8 years of age.
52. **B.**—For a very young infant, the nose examination can be done best with the child lying on his back on the table.
53. **C.**—Pale, boggy mucosa is typical of allergy while inflammation and erythema indicate infection.
54. **A.**—Trauma to the nose is often caused either by being hit or by being stuffed with a foreign body.
55. **C.**—Intermittent release of compress on both nostrils within a 10 minute period interferes with blood stoppage by pressure. If a child is having several nosebleeds a day, he should be referred to a doctor, as treatment of the cause is quite important.
56. **A.**—It is important that the fontanels will be assessed accordingly; as for example, slight pulsation of the fontanels is within normal range, but definite, great pulsations

may be an indication of intracranial pressure and should be reported immediately.
57. **A.**—The anterior fontanel is expected to close between 9 and 19 months of age.
58. **C.**—Sunken fontanels are indicative of dehydration.
59. **B.**—Infection of the scalp may also cause palpable occipital lymph nodes.
60. **C.**—Children with kwashiorkor display patches of reddish, coarse hair throughout their regular hair color.
61. **C.**—Dry, coarse hair texture may result from generalized malnutrition.
62. **B.**—If much head lag remains at this age, the nurse should suspect possible cerebral palsy or other neuromuscular deficits.
63. **B.**—Ears that do not cross the eye-occiput line are said to be low set and must be reported at once.
64. **A.**—Excessive pulsations in the neck need immediate attention and should be reported at once.
65. **C.**—Craniotabes is present in premature children and in infants suspected of rickets, syphilis, hypervitaminosis A, and hydrocephaly.
66. **D.**—Since the infant's skull bones are soft and pliable, the skull shape can be easily affected by placing the infant in one position continuously.
67. **E.**—Blepharospasm may be due to a tic or habit or may be a sign of eyestrain or irritation.
68. **H.**—Cheimosis is usually an indication of infection.
69. **A.**—Epiphora may result from an allergy or inflammation, a foreign body, a plugged lacrimal duct or exophthalmus.
70. **B.**—Congenital ptosis is often inherited and a family history should be taken.
71. **C.**—Brushfield's spots may occur in normal children but in its more striking appearance may be an indication of Down's syndrome.
72. **L.**—Short periods of nystagmus in an infant who is not yet focusing can be normal; but any continuous nystagmus, even in infants, should be referred.
73. **D.**—If there is any reason to suspect a cataract, the child should be seen by an ophthalmologist.
74. **G.**—Bitol's spots may be associated with dryness and hyperemia in the palpebral conjunctiva.
75. **I.**—The condition is an acute inflammation which causes pain in the upper lid.
76. **K.**—A clogged lacrimal duct predisposes a child to darocystitis. Massage or rubbing of the eye is contraindicated since it may spread the infection.
77. **A.**—Muscles are inserted into the scleral surface.
78. **C.**—The retina is contained in the inner nervous tunic of the eye.
79. **B.**—The fovea centralis is the central depression in the macula.
80. **C.**—Other structures for refraction within the eye proper are the zonula cilaris and crystalline lens.
81. **D.**—Percussion is not an appropriate technique for evaluating the eyes. Inspection is the primary method used and the nurse's observational skill is a most valuable tool.
82. **A.**—The reflex is otherwise known as the jaw-winking reflex.
83. **C.**—Horner's syndrome is a pupil myasthenia gravis associated with ptosis. Treacher Collins syndrome is the downward slanting of the eye.
84. **D.**—In contrast, eyelashes may be absent in premature infants, and in Treacher Collins disease lashes may be absent on the inner two-thirds of the lid.
85. **A.**—Opposite to the said condition is epiphora or excessive tearing, which may result from an allergy or inflammation and the like.
86. **B.**—The test is a light reflex test in which the room is darkened and a penlight is shone into the child's eyes. The reflection of the light should be in exactly the same position on each pupil.
87. **I.**—Syndactyly is frequently associated with premature closure of the sutures.
88. **H.**—The movement towards the medial line is called adduction.
89. **G.**—The ilium is the superior, broad, flat surface of the hip bone.
90. **B.**—Genu valgum may be normal in children between 2 and 3½ years of age.
91. **F.**—Pes cavus may be normal or a symp-

tom of Friedreich's ataxia. All children are flatfooted until they have walked for 1 to 2 years.
92. **A.**—Pes valgus refers to the entire foot turning and may be causing tibial torsion.
93. **E.**—Ankylosis is a common sequela to fractures.
94. **D.**—Polydactyly is frequently associated with Ellis-van Creveld syndrome.
95. **L.**—Tibial torsion is another name for bowleggedness.
96. **C.**—Normally, the spine curves forward and backward. If the forward and backward curves are exaggerated, they are considered pathologic.
97. **D.**—The skin has nothing to do with the production of Vitamin K. It is associated with the production of Vitamin D.
98. **B.**—In contrast, the dermis is the vascular part of the skin.
99. **D.**—The stratum basale represents the deepest part of the skin.
100. **B.**—The active growth stage of the hair is called the anagen stage.
101. **B.**—When the total serum bilirubin reaches 5 mg/100 ml in the newborn he is visibly jaundiced.
102. **C.**—Jaundice is best seen in true sunlight by looking at the sclera, mucous membranes, or skin.
103. **D.**—Sometimes one-half of the newborn's body is red and the other half pale (Harlequin sign); this is not a pathologic condition and usually is transitory.
104. **D.**—Normal, hydrated skin rises with the pinch but quickly falls when released. Dry, dehydrated skin will remain in the pinched position.
105. **C.**—Scaliness may occur on several parts of the body. Vitamin A deficiency, *not* vitamin C, may also cause rough and dry skin.
106. **C.**—Seborrhea is no cause for concern but if left unattended will predispose infections.
107. **A.**—Milia is very common during the hot season.
108. **B.**—Milia does not need elaborate treatment unless complicated with secondary infections. Just keep baby from sweating but when sweating occurs, let it dry quickly.
109. **C.**—Port wine stain is present at birth as a flat, reddish capillary lesion and is most common around the scalp and face.
110. **D.**—The said conditions may be indicative of such diseases as hemophilia, purpuras or leukemia or child abuse.
111. **H.**—Cavernous hemangiomas may be found on any portion of the skin and usually disappear spontaneously.
112. **M.**—They are staphylococcal infections which are commonly found in eyelids, eyelashes and eyebrows.
113. **I.**—Normal, hydrated skin rises with the pinch but quickly falls when released.
114. **A.**—Macules are seen in rubeola, rubella, scarlet fever, and roseola infantum.
115. **F.**—This hair generally disappears before or shortly after birth.
116. **E.**—Pustules are seen in impetigo, acne, and staphylococcal infections.
117. **D.**—It is believed that the vernix caseosa protects the skin and the current practice is to leave it on rather than vigorously scrubbing it off during the initial care of the newborn.
118. **J.**—Vitiligo may appear as irregular patches or white spots in what is ordinarily a melanotic skin.
119. **K.**—Xanthomas are local accumulations of fatty material and usually dissolve in a few weeks.
120. **C.**—Pruritus, like pain, is a highly subjective symptom.
121. **C.**—Wheals appear and disappear quickly; they are seen in mosquito bites, hives, and urticaria.
122. **B.**—A good example of such condition is a scrape or scratch.
123. **A.**—It is commonly known as a blister.
124. **D.**—The condition is due to chronic scratching or rubbing.
125. **B.**—Papules are seen in ringworm and psoriasis.
126. **C.**—Ulcers are very hard to treat.
127. **B.**—Sweat is not seen sooner unless the infant has brain irritation, a sympathetic nervous system disorder, or a mother who is a chronic morphine user.
128. **B.**—Good natural lighting is the most important equipment for skin examination

with the techniques of inspection and palpation.
129. **A.**—Percussion is a technique used for determining the density of various parts of the body involving organs underneath the skin.
130. **D.**—In addition, cooling baths during hot weather is helpful. Excess skin folds should be carefully rinsed and thoroughly dried.
131. **C.**—Such procedure only pastes the scales down, giving the illusion that the dermatitis is disappearing.
132. **B.**—Diaper rash is produced on the skin by the interaction of urea and bacteria which vastly multiply in diaper areas covered by tight-fitting diapers and plastic pants.
133. **D.**—An important health point to be learned by mothers is to change diapers as soon as they become wet.
134. **D.**—Soiled diapers should be soaked in a solution of wet borax and thoroughly rinsed. The baby should always be kept dry.
135. **B.**—The stomach is an organ of the gastro-intestinal system.
136. **C.**—The nodes to be palpated in the head are: posterior, auricular, preoccipital, superficial cervical, submental, submandibular, mandibular, parotid, and inferior deep cervical.
137. **D.**—In acute infections, nodes will frequently appear tender, warm and large.
138. **B.**—The inguinal nodes are easily palpated along the crease separating the thigh from the abdomen.
139. **A.**—Scalp infections, rubella and pediculosis also cause occipital nodes to swell.
140. **C.**—The head, neck, inguinal, axillary and arm areas are a must for boys and girls; the breast is a must only for girls.
141. **A.**—This type of node is generally normal in moderate numbers or it may be a sign of past infections.
142. **C.**—Signs of dyspnea are restlessness, apprehension, retractions, nasal flaring, cyanosis, and clubbing.
143. **I.**—Scoliosis may be pathologic and should always be a cause for concern.
144. **L.**—Subcutaneous crepitus may be discovered on palpation which may indicate gas gangrene or subcutaneous emphysema.
145. **F.**—Bradypnea may be due to brain tumors or opiate poisoning.
146. **A.**—Alkalotic breathing on the other hand is diminished in depth and is slow and shallow.
147. **B.**—The vital capacity for an adult is 3700 ml and less for a growing child.
148. **H.**—Biot's breathing is a very serious pattern of respiration.
149. **G.**—Cheyne-Stokes respiration is a common sign of impending death.
150. **E.**—The condition is commonly known as hump back.
151. **J.**—This is performed by coordination of the chest muscles to expand and decrease the volume of the chest cavity.
152. **A.**—The diaphragm is a large musculofibrous membrane, the cranial surface being convex and the caudal, concave.
153. **B.**—The structure is a part of the lower respiratory tract with its superior portion divided into the anterior, middle and posterior mediastinum.
154. **C.**—In health, the pleura are simply two membranes lying together. In illness, the area of the cavity increases with air or fluid separating the membranes.
155. **D.**—The larynx, otherwise called the voice box, is contained in the trachea.
156. **D.**—Inflammation of the costochondral junction forms a series of palpable bumps similar to rosary beads, hence the term rachitic rosary.
157. **B.**—A barrel chest is usually accompanied by kyphosis.
158. **D.**—When marked deviations are seen in the respiratory rates expected of certain age groups, they should be a cause for concern.
159. **A.**—The transition to costal respiration is gradual until about 7 years of age, at which time it should be predominantly costal. A very young child should be closely observed for dyspnea if he breathes costally as for an older child who primarily breathes abdominally.
160. **D.**—In children of all ages, breath sounds can be classified into three basic categories; vesicular, visceral, and bronchial or tubular breath sounds.
161. **H.**—The possibility of a heart block should be considered if S_1 is constantly changing

in intensity and is accompanied by bradycardia.
162. **E.**—Inflammation of the muscular layer of the heart is called myocarditis.
163. **B.**—The first heart sound is designated S₁ and indicates the systolic part of the cardiac cycle.
164. **A.**—A nurse should refer all murmurs to the physician and let him distinguish between innocent and organic types.
165. **J.**—The bundle of His is a bundle of nerve fibers travelling from the atrioventricular node to the apex.
166. **C.**—The apical area is a very important one and is located at the fifth intercostal space in the midclavicular line in adults and children over approximately 8 years of age.
167. **L.**—The sign is always abnormal and can be associated with organic heart disease, rheumatic fever, thyrotoxicosis or other serious illnesses.
168. **I.**—This type of pulse is often accompanied by capillary pulsations of the fingernail.
169. **F.**—In the pulmonic area, any thrill radiating to the left side of the neck should be referred to the doctor as this may be a sign of pulmonary stenosis.
170. **D.**—The opening snap occurs soon after S₂ in the third to fourth left intercostal space.
171. **B.**—Five of every thousand infants are born with a congenital heart defect. The incidence is two to three times higher in premature infants.
172. **A.**—The peak age of incidence for rheumatic fever is from 5 to 15 years of age, however, a careful heart evaluation should always be done on the 2-week follow-up visit after streptococcal infections.
173. **C.**—For the newborn, the normal pulse rate is 70–170; infants, 80–160; school age, 70–110 beats per minute.
174. **C.**—Salmonella infection is associated with a fever accompanied by a slow pulse, although fever ordinarily increases the pulse rate.
175. **B.**—Normally, this is about 20 to 50 mm Hg throughout childhood. An unusually wide pulse pressure may be due to an abnormally high systolic reading or an abnormally low diastolic reading.
176. **A.**—An abnormally low diastolic reading is usually associated with serious heart diseases such as patent ductus arteriosus and aortic regurgitation, hence its clinical significance.
177. **D.**—Closure of the semilunar valve causes the second heart sound (S₂). It reflects diastole and is the "dub" of the "lub-dub."
178. **F.**—On the posterior end of the stomach is the pyloric valve which allows the stomach to empty into the duodenum.
179. **H.**—Just as a Cullen's sign may occur with intra-abdominal hemorrhage, a nodular umbilicus may be a sign of abdominal cancer.
180. **L.**—The duodenum empties its contents into the jejunum, which is the vascular portion of the small intestines and contains large villi.
181. **J.**—Organomegaly, tenderness, or masses are all important signs that should be carefully observed in the examination.
182. **D.**—Glistening, thick skin or bulging of the flanks may indicate ascites.
183. **C.**—Spider nevi appears as spider-shaped reddened areas with a central arteriole and several extending rays.
184. **A.**—On abdominal palpation, a plastic feel to the mass will be noted by the examiner in megacolon cases.
185. **B.**—The mark appears as reddish blue, bluish purple, or greenish brown with no history of trauma.
186. **E.**—Striae should be noted on the abdomen as well as on the shoulders, thighs and breasts.
187. **G.**—Observation for possible hernias must be a part of every abdominal examination for children. Inguinal hernias are fairly common in children and seldom cause pain, particularly the direct type.
188. **A.**—Peristalsis and pressure are two types of muscular activity within the stomach. Pressures force the food into contact with the stomach wall and gastric juices.
189. **B.**—The jejunum is found in the umbilical and left portions of the abdominal wall.
190. **D.**—The liver weighs 1.2 to 1.4 kg and is soft and highly vascular.

191. **C.**—Insulin is secreted by the islands of Langerhans.
192. **B.**—The spleen is a highly variable organ in size and function.
193. **C.**—Such a sign may also indicate duodenal ulcer, malrotation of the bowel, urinary tract infection, duodenal stenosis or gastrointestinal allergy.
194. **B.**—The sign is otherwise called Sister Joseph's nodule.
195. **A.**—There is no general agreement as to treatment of hernias.
196. **D.**—The first three choices are indicative of umbilical infection and this can be quite dangerous in a young infant since infection can readily spread to the peritoneum via the open arteries. This may eventually cause septicemia.
197. **C.**—In adolescence, girls will reveal a triangular distribution of hair in the pubic area while the boys will reveal a diamond shaped distribution.
198. **B.**—It appears as a small bulge adjacent and medial to the femoral artery by about 2 finger breadths.
199. **A.**—Inflamed spleen may reveal friction rubbing and congenital abnormalities of umbilical vein may reveal venous hum.
200. **D.**—A light touch should be employed.
201. **A.**—The two components are the brain (encephalon) and spinal cord (medulla spinalis).
202. **C.**—The ganglia are either sensory or autonomic.
203. **B.**—The cortex is divided into 11 areas thought to control specific functions.
204. **D.**—The cerebrospinal fluid flows in the subarachnoid space.
205. **A.**—Broca's area is the speech region, thus controlling the ability to articulate speech.
206. **C.**—Unless it is necessary, deep pressure pain should not be used, since rapport with the child will frequently be lost.
207. **D.**—The important clues for a young child's state of consciousness are primarily motor rather than verbal. Severe avitaminosis is not always associated with extreme drowsiness.
208. **A.**—Remote memory refers to memory which holds for longer periods of time.
209. **C.**—Children under 5 years of age are developmentally too immature to be able to compare weights.
210. **B.**—Stereogenetic disorders are associated with cerebral palsy, peripheral neuropathy, parietal lobe disorders, or posterior column diseases.
211. **A.**—The child closes his eyes and must tell the examiner whether his finger is up or down.
212. **C.**—Auditory agnosia originates in the lateral and superior portions of the temporal lobe.
213. **D.**—The child is then asked to identify familiar odors.
214. **C.**—The trigeminal and facial nerves are the fifth cranial nerve and the seventh cranial nerve respectively.
215. **B.**—Balance and coordination may be reflected in the quality of skilled activity a child is able to do using a developmental screening tool.
216. **A.**—Lesions in the cerebellar lobe may cause staggering and falling.
217. **D.**—After 2 months, extension gradually becomes more pronounced following a cephalocaudal pattern.
218. **B.**—Spasticity is among the earliest signs of cerebral palsy.
219. **C.**—Another useful test is for the examiner to flex the infant's legs onto his abdomen and then release them quickly. In an infant with cerebral palsy, the legs may extend quickly and then abduct to a scissoring position.
220. **A.**—Other aspects of the newborn's position are influenced by his position in utero.
221. **D.**—The frog position may be normal in a breech position but it should call for further neurologic evaluation if in a vertex position.
222. **D.**—The floppy infant will have greater head lag than normal plus a floppy, lumpy trunk and dangling arms and legs.
223. **B.**—This type of movement is usually not demonstrated until about the 18th month.
224. **A.**—Plantar flexion of foot demonstrates positive Achilles reflex.
225. **C.**—Before the child has begun to walk, the normal response is fanning of the toes, particularly of the big toe, and the abnormal response is a plantar flexion. After

Health Maintenance and Promotion 99

225. (cont.) the child has begun to walk, the reverse is true.
226. **C.**—The normal response is an incurving of the toes toward the stimulus (plantar flexion).
227. **A.**—The responses to all the aforenoted reflexes are evaluated in the same way as the Babinski reflex.
228. **A.**—The nurse should worry about a child who displays the tonic neck reflex particularly before 2 to 3 months of age, and who seems "locked" in the "fencer position."
229. **B.**—The situation would already be of clinical significance if it were seen persistently at 4 to 5 months.
230. **A.**—The response is less vigorous during the first 2 days of life and if it is absent later, the baby should be suspected of being in a depressed state, particularly if barbiturates have been used by the mother.
231. **D.**—Sucking is less intense in the first 3 or 4 days. Barbiturates transmitted in the breast milk will depress sucking.
232. **C.**—It is expected to be present from birth to 3 or 4 months. If it lasts longer than 6 months, it should definitely be considered abnormal.
233. **D.**—Damage to the medulla oblongata often causes death.
234. **C.**—The hypothalamus is composed of gray matter and is located inferior to the thalamus.
235. **H.**—The thalamus is a large mass of gray matter forming the lateral wall of the third ventricle.
236. **A.**—Disorders of proprioception primarily reflect abnormalities in the cerebellum.
237. **E.**—Each neuron has one axon but may have several dendrites.
238. **B.**—The pons is a ventral protuberance of the brainstem.
239. **F.**—Motor aphasia can result from damage to this area.
240. **J.**—Impulses are received through the dendrites.
241. **G.**—Impulses leave the cell body through the axon where they can be transmitted through a synapse to the dendrite of the next neuron.
242. **I.**—The parietal area is indeed vital to the control and integration of human behavior.
243. **A.**—Anxiety could either be therapeutic or pathologic, as the case may be, the cause of which always remains obscure to the individual.
244. **C.**—Anxiety is nonspecific. One's emotional response seems to have little relevance to actual outside stimuli.
245. **C.**—Such treatment would render the nurse blind and deaf to the subtle signs and symptoms of emotional stress display.
246. **C.**—Aggressive behavior is very easy to identify because it is so universal in dimension and it is overtly expressed in children. The cause is fairly easy to identify but the *why* of the cause may be more difficult to establish.
247. **D.**—Aggressive acts are frequently tinged with hostility but *not always* associated with it.
248. **B.**—As the child learns to handle his aggression in socially acceptable ways, he becomes a happier child since he also experiences a diminution in his need for attention and affection fulfillment.
249. **D.**—Through play, the child learns to express his feelings, whether love or anger.
250. **C.**—The use of musical toys is not too appropriate for helping release aggressive feelings since it does not call for active physical involvement.
251. **C.**—Signal anxiety sets the person in a state of readiness.
252. **A.**—An anxious child would hardly be expected to be excessively quiet and withdrawn for he has just too much energy to contend with.
253. **D.**—Withdrawal would hardly help a child work out his fear and anxiety.
254. **B.**—The child tears off on a binge of general wild behavior and destruction in a diffuse way.
255. **A.**—Fortunately, repression happens only in extreme cases.
256. **C.**—Clinging to fantasies of power, force, and indestructibility is beneficial if the child is faced with anxiety rather than with reality-determined fears.
257. **B.**—Under such a condition, the ego of the child seems to have been damaged.

258. **A.**—The toddler shows that he has a mind and a will of his own.
259. **B.**—"No" is an easy sound to make and he may use it for personal pleasure rather than for expression of a negative feeling.
260. **B.**—The toddler who has been given gradual independence which brings pleasurable results develops a sense of self-reliance and adequacy.
261. **B.**—The toddler generally enjoys parallel play best.
262. **C.**—It is very important to help a child establish a strong self-image.
263. **D.**—The nurse should try to exploit as much environmental resources as possible to help the child develop socially, which is an important aspect of his total personality development.
264. **A.**—The aggression of the boy towards his father has been introjected to himself, causing him to exhibit personality deviations via accession.
265. **A.**—Parents must be supportive of the adolescent's gradual emancipation from them and family.
266. **A.**—The child's sense of initiative must be encouraged throughout childhood and youth.
267. **C.**—Many children shamed beyond endurance may be in a chronic mood to express defiance.
268. **A.**—It is important for the nurse to understand that people are generally not comfortable about exposing their inner self.
269. **C.**—Thus, the importance of the nurse is to assist the family, assess the crisis situation, and help them out before they get overwhelmed by the crisis situation.
270. **B.**—The new force drives him to his peers. His sexual feelings do not necessarily drive him to the sexual act, although some physical expressions of affection are common.
271. **D.**—Prejudiced groups maintain a closed system.
272. **C.**—Sensory deprivation is only a part of environmental deprivation, although the two terms are often used interchangeably.
273. **A.**—It is generally accepted that the family is a basic factor that can provide a child the adult-nurturing process essential to a healthy development in infancy and childhood.
274. **D.**—Spitz and Bowlby, in their individual works as early as 1946 and 1951 respectively, both strongly made awareness of the problem of environmental deprivation and child development the concern of health professionals.
275. **B.**—Infants suffering from maternal deprivation are very much lacking emotional affection.
276. **C.**—The child is in a fit of crying during the protest stage, then gets quiet and subdued (despair) and finally would seem to be unaffected by what is going on around him, including his mother (denial).
277. **B.**—This age group has been observed to be virtually defenseless when faced with a painful stimulus.
278. **A.**—Knowing the vulnerability of this group of children, the nurse and other health workers must be alert for manifestation of deprivations.
279. **D.**—Pathologic anxiety, otherwise known as traumatic anxiety, immobilizes the individual's personal resources.
280. **B.**—The signal type of anxiety plays an important role in growth and development.
281. **B.**—A child who has suffered from maternal deprivation shortly after birth could not be expected to seek out contact with adults, not even the mother, since he had not really learned to relate with any significant other.
282. **C.**—If a child is being placed continuously in the same playpen, then he is likely to get bored and therefore would not be sufficiently stimulated.
283. **D.**—The infant is already under a physical and emotional strain from his illness, therefore weaning him at this time would only aggravate the situation.
284. **D.**—In the first situation, the child seems helpless in view of an onrush of impulse intensity, and in the second situation, he seems helpless when confronted with increasing fear, discomfort and aggression produced by even mildly "frustrating" situations.
285. **A.**—Abrupt completion of the weaning

Health Maintenance and Promotion

process would likely be traumatic and frustrating to the infant. Under this condition, the infant is unlikely to seek contact with surrounding adults.
286. **D.**—Suicide occurs most often in the 15–19 year age group. It is surpassed only by accidents, cancer, and homicides as a cause of death.
287. **D.**—Many such adolescents act out their feelings through drug abuse, alcoholism and sexual promiscuity.
288. **B.**—A young child is much more vulnerable to traumatic anxiety because he has limited experience to prepare him for, and little understanding and ability to cope with, threatening situations.
289. **B.**—Older children may become verbally aggressive.
290. **C.**—The child may become an observer from a safe distance or he may actually withdraw within himself.
291. **A.**—Frustration is a necessary ingredient of maturation. The child who never meets frustration in his youth would have real difficulty in coping with the problems in adulthood.
292. **C.**—The child's "goodness" is his own worst enemy and should be a real cause of concern to those caring for him.
293. **D.**—In regressive behavior, the child assumes behavior similar to the earlier secure period in which he felt his needs were met.
294. **A.**—Both tests are aimed at discovering excessive heterophoria or strabismus. The Snellen test and Ishihara color blindness test require that the child must have the ability to recognize basic forms and color.
295. **D.**—The other three conditions cause dilatation of pupils.
296. **B.**—Pupils constrict when focusing on a nearby object.
297. **B.**—Permanent color of the iris will be manifested in 50% of children by 6 months.
298. **C.**—The otoscope is used for examining the ears.
299. **A.**—When using an ophthalmoscope, the examiner must see to it that the child will hold his eyes still and that the evaluation will be started at a distance of about 12 inches from the patient.
300. **D.**—Test should be carried out at the standard 20 foot distance.
301. **B.**—Both tests are very simple to administer and mothers could easily be taught to administer either one.
302. **A.**—Her acuity is recorded as 20/30 because the 30 foot line was the last line from which she could read four out of six symbols correctly.
303. **D.**—Cataracts are opacities of the lens. Causes of cataracts include maternal rubella, galactosemia, hypoparathyroidism, or trauma.
304. **B.**—Early detection of amblyopia could prevent further loss of vision in the unused eye. Testing each eye separately is essential.
305. **C.**—Strabismus is the most common cause of one-eye blindness in children. Strabismus can usually be prevented. The muscles of the two eyes fail to keep the eyes in alignment.
306. **D.**—Vomiting just before going to school can very well be a symptom of psychological problems. The child may simply detest going to school.
307. **B.**—Frequent complaints of headache may indicate brain tumor or brain infections, e.g., encephalitis.
308. **D.**—The results of the Snellen test are expressed in a fraction, the numerator indicating the distance of the child from the chart and the denominator the smallest line read correctly. Normal vision is 20/20 in the Snellen test.
309. **A.**—Refer pupils *only after* a second screening has been made. Referrals on the basis of one screening only have too frequently been found to result in error.
310. **B.**—Postpone the screening if child does not have his glasses the day of the screening.
311. **C.**—Color blindness presents a particular problem for young children, particularly in relation to school, because many of the cues encountered in the academic setting depend upon the ability to distinguish colors.
312. **B.**—Visual acuity can reliably be screened by the use of the Snellen test.

313. **D.**—Training paraprofessional workers for screening test administration is not one of the purposes of a screening program.
314. **A.**—Refractive errors cannot be screened out by the use of the Snellen test.
315. **D.**—Loss of less than 30 db in any frequency is acceptable hearing. Concern about this finding occurs with the presence of pathological conditions pertaining to the ear.
316. **A.**—Vision defects are among the most common handicapping conditions of childhood and effective screening is of special importance since many of these problems are remedial.
317. **C.**—Heterophoria is otherwise called latent squint.
318. **B.**—This criterion is, however, not universally accepted.
319. **D.**—Sometimes, despite adequate preparation, a few children are untestable by any of the recommended methods.
320. **A.**—The Draw-a-Man test is one of the tests to assess intelligence of children over four or five years of age.
321. **B.**—The hematocrit value averages between 36 and 38 percent by five years of age.
322. **C.**—About 9% of American Negroes are heterozygous for hemoglobin S and perhaps 0.2 to 0.3 percent have sickle cell disease.
323. **D.**—In many states the PKU. test is required by law and the American Academy of Pediatrics has recommended routine urine testing for screening galactosemia in neonates.
324. **D.**—The incidence of pica is extremely high in children.
325. **B.**—Lead poisoning is treatable even in the clinical stage as long as encephalopathy has not yet developed.
326. **A.**—The child between 1 and 3 years of age is in the exploratory stage and tends to put everything in his mouth. Obviously, lead is more readily ingested in this age group than in any other group.
327. **C.**—It requires venipuncture, hence, impractical for screening purposes.
328. **B.**—Tuberculosis remains an important disease in the United States especially among the urban indigent population and particularly in children under five years of age.
329. **B.**—The parents should be provided with a small photograph showing typical reactions if they are to be asked to read it and send in the report.
330. **D.**—The said children usually have adequate sensory acuity, however, their academic achievement is below what would be expected by the composite of their I.Q. score, age, educational opportunity, health and cultural opportunities.
331. **B.**—An important aspect to consider is the fact that the subaverage intellectual functioning originated during the developmental period.
332. **C.**—Educable children can generally respond to traditional education in reading, writing and arithmetic.
333. **C.**—A child with an I.Q. score of approximately 30 to 49 is trainable.
334. **D.**—As many as 75 to 85% of all retarded children may be classified in category D.
335. **A.**—Standard deviations of I.Q. scores are used as points, e.g., the borderline mentally retardate falls within S.D. −1 to −2; Stanford-Binet scores 83 to 68.
336. **B.**—It is best to have the mentally retarded children in special classes by virtue of their special needs, however, the experiences planned should be similar to those of all other children.
337. **A.**—All of the said children correspond with the educational classification of custodial.
338. **B.**—This group is estimated to include 13.59% of the total population.
339. **D.**—The trainable mental retardate in a supervised setting can gain skills that will enable him to make meaningful contributions and limited earnings.
340. **A.**—The child who has a marked hearing loss requires amplified levels of conversation in order to hear.
341. **B.**—The purpose of the hearing conservation program is to detect the student with a heavy loss as soon as possible, in order to provide for adequate follow-up procedures and make appropriate adjustments in the student's school program.

342. **D.**—The aforenoted factors should always be kept in mind when developing a screening test program.
343. **A.**—The Bureau of Education for the Handicapped estimated that 0.5% of all school-age children have some hearing loss which interferes with education and learning.
344. **D.**—Studies have demonstrated that children and youth who are continuously exposed to loud noise, such as blaring radios and television, suffer from varying degrees of hearing impairment.
345. **B.**—If the child is over 3 years, the auricle is pulled up and back in order to facilitate the passage of the fluid onto the drum.
346. **B.**—The older child will complain of severe, sharp pain in the ear, but the infant often has no great discomfort and may cry very little.
347. **D.**—Studies have shown that accidental injury to the ear, noise damage, and presence of foreign bodies in the ear canal are among the common causes of hearing loss during childhood.
348. **D.**—There is presently no satisfactory way to restore hearing loss due to nerve impairment.
349. **C.**—Constant association with hearing peers and family members is important for optimal adjustment of these children.
350. **C.**—Loud noises may be heard at some distance.
351. **B.**—A person may have a hearing level of 26 db and still evidence no hearing loss.
352. **B.**—It is important to retest the child another time and day to rule out possible factors that may have biased the findings.
353. **D.**—Examination of the tympanic membrane is of utmost importance in any hearing assessment.
354. **A.**—Any change in color deserves further study.
355. **C.**—If fluid is contained in the middle ear, the tympanic membrane will not move, or if it does, it moves in a sticky fashion.
356. **B.**—Conductive hearing loss is indicated audiometrically by a difference of 10 decibles or more between the air conduction and bone conduction thresholds.
357. **C.**—Accumulation of ear wax blocks the canal, preventing sound waves from reaching the eardrum.
358. **B.**—The pinna is otherwise called the auricle.
359. **A.**—Thus, any infection in the middle ear can easily spread into the brain structures because of its close proximity.
360. **C.**—The head of the stapes connects to the incus and the flat base lies close to the inner ear.
361. **D.**—The tympanic membrane is a part of the middle ear.
362. **C.**—In infants, the ear is pulled down since the canal curves upward.
363. **A.**—The eustachian tube serves as a pressure equalizing device so that pressures on both sides of the eardrum will be the same. The tube also provides a convenient pathway for infection from nose and throat to middle ear.
364. **D.**—The site for lobar pneumonia is not as close to the middle ear as it is for the aforenoted conditions.
365. **A.**—Fortunately, with the current use of antibiotics, mastoiditis is no longer a very dangerous complication, as the infection could now be readily checked.
366. **B.**—In otosclerosis, a spongy type of bone grows around the window linking the middle and inner ears, causing a fixation of the stirrup.
367. **C.**—Stapedectomy is the partial or complete removal of the stapes, the innermost of the three bones lying behind the tympanic membrane.
368. **D.**—Most congenital ear problems result from damage to the cochlea which may be hereditary or acquired during the gestation period.
369. **D.**—Exposure to sudden loud noise may cause permanent damage to hearing; vascular disturbances may cause heavy hearing impairment by depriving the cochlea of oxygen; measles, mumps and meningitis may cause destruction of the nerve tissue within the cochlea.
370. **A.**—Once a sensorineural type of tissue is damaged, it remains damaged, since such tissue cannot regenerate.
371. **C.**—The audiometer provides a simple, reliable, and effective means of screening

children with hearing impairments from those with normal hearing.
372. **C.**—Children would probably have some difficulty pronouncing rarely used words because of the lack of practice.
373. **A.**—Mouth breathing should be a cause of concern especially if associated with earache or discharge from one or both ears.
374. **C.**—A reading of −10 db means 10 db better than the average normal ear's acuity; +10 db means 10 db worse than the average.
375. **A.**—In most school surveys, between 5 and 10% of the enrollment will fail to pass the screening test. If more than 10% fail, any one of the four factors or more may be operating.
376. **D.**—The threshold at each of the test frequencies should be charted on an audiogram. If there is any difference in acuity between the two ears, the better ear should be tested first.
377. **B.**—The data is based on the *1964 International Standards Organization Reference.*
378. **A.**—A loss in either ear of 20 db or more at 2 or more frequencies or a loss of 30 db or more at any single frequency is considered to be clinically significant.
379. **C.**—Care must be taken not to cause undue concern on the part of the parents particularly when the child's hearing impairment is only borderline.
380. **A.**—The said agency also maintains a registry of approved clinical programs in speech and hearing.
381. **C.**—Early dental care enables the dentist to discover and correct defects in the earliest stages. Periodic check-ups permit the dentist to observe the child's dental growth pattern and detect early symptoms of diseases. Prompt action will prevent undue pain, serious complication and loss of teeth.
382. **A.**—Thirty-two teeth make up the full set of permanent teeth.
383. **A.**—Records show that the loss of deciduous molars usually occurs between 10½ and 12 years of age.
384. **C.**—Upper deciduous incisors usually erupt between 6 and 8 months of age.
385. **B.**—The permanent second molars erupt by the twelfth year and are usually completed by the sixteenth year.
386. **C.**—On the contrary, twenty is a complete set of deciduous teeth.
387. **B.**—Earlier eruption of teeth in girls than in boys consequently subjects girls' teeth to longer exposure to attack by caries.
388. **A.**—Caries are a very common health problem and should be checked for at every visit. However, there is no evidence to show that approximately 30% of 2-year-old children have one or more carious teeth.
389. **A.**—Such measure permits fluoridated water to be made available to large numbers of people at a relatively low cost.
390. **D.**—To help families in their decision making, the facts, alternative choices, and possible consequences of each alternative should be made available.
391. **A.**—Individual children differ in their response to different approaches, and the needs of the child must necessarily be determined in developing an educational program.
392. **B.**—It is basically important to determine whether the child's learning problem is general or specific. If the child's failure is related to general inadequacy in functioning, he will most likely be identified as having some type of retardation.
393. **D.**—D.P.T. immunization, commonly known as the triple vaccine, is one of the routine immunizations required for all infants in the United States. Routine smallpox vaccination is no longer recommended.
394. **B.**—Pertussis vaccine is not necessary for children over 6 years.
395. **C.**—The triple antigen vaccine is composed of diphtheria and tetanus toxoids combined with pertussis vaccine.
396. **A.**—The Salk polio vaccine is suitable for breast-fed as well as bottle-fed infants.
397. **A.**—Priority is given to preschool and elementary school ages.
398. **D.**—Mumps vaccine may be given with measles-rubella combined vaccine.
399. **B.**—Passively transmitted maternal antibodies may prevent adequate active immunity in the infant.

Health Maintenance and Promotion

400. **D.**—Parental consent is not a crucial factor in the administration of tuberculin tests.
401. **A.**—An acutely ill child should not be given immunization materials. Pertussis vaccine should not be given to any infant or child who has a history of convulsions.
402. **C.**—The child should be subcutaneously injected with .5 ml of tetanus toxoid to provide immediate increase in immunity.
403. **A.**—Such recommendation is a compromise. Some doctors may not recommend starting the immunization until the twelfth week of life.
404. **C.**—On the other hand, infants do have adequate passively acquired protection against diphtheria and tetanus for up to 6 months, if their mothers are immune.
405. **A.**—Prolongation of the intervals, while it may not result in lower antibody levels, delays protection against the specific disease.
406. **B.**—Pertussis vaccine is the least effective component of D.P.T., nevertheless, current studies show that current preparations have made the disease less severe and have reduced the attack rates among susceptibles after home exposures from 90 to 15 percent.
407. **A.**—The Schick test is a toxoid sensitivity test.
408. **C.**—The scapular area or the popliteal fossa may also be used.
409. **C.**—There is a danger of contaminating the vaccination with fecal matter. In any case cleansing the skin with acetone rather than alcohol prevents inactivation of the virus and results in fewer "no-take" reactions.
410. **B.**—In the presence of an epidemic or in the event of unusual exposure, smallpox vaccination should be repeated.
411. **D.**—So far its use with children has been largely confined to cases of exposure to measles.
412. **D.**—The vaccination should always be repeated.
413. **A.**—The reaction site should be observed one week after immunization before signing certificates of successful vaccination.
414. **A.**—Refer to preceding explanation.
415. **B.**—In countries with a high morbidity for measles, the measles immunization should be started between ages 6 and 9 months with a booster dose at 15 to 18 months.
416. **D.**—Positive reactors to tuberculin tests should be placed on anti-tuberculosis therapy before giving the measles vaccine.
417. **C.**—Only *killed* vaccines should be used for children with altered immune responses.
418. **A.**—BCG and influenza are needed only by certain high risk groups. Smallpox vaccination is *now* optional.
419. **B.**—The administration of the oral live poliomyelitis vaccine is the simplest of all immunizing procedures. It is made up of 2 drops of freshly reconstituted vaccine dropped into the mouth or fed on a small lump of sugar.
420. **D.**—Explanation is an important part of health supervision. The mother should know what to expect. Also, she should be given a record of immunization and the importance of her keeping it up to date should be emphasized.
421. **D.**—If the child seems mildly anxious, it is a good practice to do the injection first in order to get it over with. With a very young child, the injection may be best given last.
422. **B.**—When using combined precipitated or absorbed toxoid vaccine mixtures, the injection should be given intramuscularly and the muscle should be injected only once during the series.
423. **D.**—It is quite important *not* to massage the site if only to permit best local reaction. Backflow during withdrawal of the needle should be prevented.
424. **C.**—Antibodies to fight off specific infections are readily provided by the gamma globulin, thus the body system is a passive recipient of the immunization process.
425. **B.**—Under such a condition, it may be advisable to give typhoid fever vaccine even as early as the first year.
426. **B.**—Mumps, in mature males, may be complicated by orchitis which can lead to sterility. Rubella in women, during the first trimester of pregnancy, may cause congenital malformation of the fetus.
427. **D.**—In addition, local soreness may be relieved by cold compresses.

428. **B.**—When the reaction is "no-take" the child should be revaccinated observing proper technique. Make sure that the vaccine is not composed of dead virus.
429. **B.**—The redness develops in a few days and lasts a week or 10 days.
430. **D.**—Never put any type of drug over the vaccinated area.
431. **D.**—Passive immunity is administered by the use of gamma globulin.
432. **D.**—Each health center must keep a schedule for active immunization and vaccination as recommended by the American Academy of Pediatrics.
433. **C.**—D.P.T. stands for the alum-precipitated diphtheria and tetanus toxoids and the pertussis vaccine.
434. **A.**—There are practically no reactions to this preparation.
435. **D.**—If a booster dose is to be given, it is for purposes of providing immediate increase in immunity.
436. **A.**—About 50 cal/lb per day (110 cal/kg) is required in the first year. The total requirement increases by 100 cal for each year of age.
437. **C.**—Water is necessary for metabolic transport, regulation of body temperature, ionic equilibrium, and a variety of cellular functions. Concerning water, the average infant requires approximately 15% of body weight per day.
438. **C.**—Carbohydrates are also the best source of energy.
439. **A.**—Breast milk contains 7% carbohydrates, while cow's milk has only 4.5%.
440. **A.**—Both kinds of milk contain 20 C/oz and 3.5% fat.
441. **B.**—The curds in human milk are soft and flocculent, hence digestion is more rapid than it is in cow's milk.
442. **D.**—Iron deficiency causes anemia.
443. **B.**—The older child needs 2 to 2½ gm of proteins per kg per day.
444. **A.**—Carbohydrates are derived from starchy foods.
445. **D.**—Otherwise, the current use of commercial formula preparations could permit even more convenience than breast-feeding.
446. **A.**—Cow's milk contains 3.5% proteins while human milk has only 1.5%.
447. **C.**—Phenylalanine is an essential amino acid present in all natural protein foods. Other foods permitted on a low phenylalanine diet are sugar, cereals and vegetables.
448. **A.**—Strict adherence to the dietary regimen cannot be overemphasized. The nurse can discuss with the mother what foods to buy and various recipes for gluten-free foods.
449. **B.**—A friendly atmosphere and enjoyment of the meal are the best aids to appetite.
450. **D.**—It means that the adolescent should receive up to 60 gm of protein a day to maintain a positive nitrogen balance.
451. **C.**—Boys, in general, are more interested in physical activity than are girls, hence they require more calories than do girls.
452. **A.**—He also needs at least 2 to 4 glasses of milk to provide calcium.
453. **B.**—Eating problems relate more to time of eating and manner of eating than to content and amount of food consumed. Then, school children are generally disciplined in table manners.
454. **A.**—Proteins yield ions to maintain the acid-base balance.
455. **D.**—Specifically, magnesium is crucial to not only bone formation and enzyme production but also for neuromuscular tissues.
456. **C.**—Water is also necessary for metabolic transport.
457. **B.**—Carbohydrates are also required for production of antibodies.
458. **D.**—It has been proven that the mineral fluorides, in particular, prevent dental caries.
459. **A.**—A number of amino acids are essential for new tissue formation and a lack of any one of these results in a negative nitrogen balance.
460. **D.**—The average diet contains many times more than the daily requirement of chlorides.
461. **C.**—Calcium requirements vary with total size and increase during periods of growth.
462. **B.**—The clinical features may be found singly or in combination, reflecting increased capillary fragility, gingival changes, or frank scurvy.
463. **A.**—The nutritional requirements during the school age remain ultimately greater

than in the mature years because of the relatively greater rate of the growth and developmental processes occurring in the school years.
464. **A.**—Appetite is a conditioned response and is not necessarily associated with physiologic hunger.
465. **C.**—Servings should be small. It is more appetizing to the child to have small portions presented. Above all, the child gets satisfied and feels accomplishment at finishing manageable portions.
466. **D.**—The overall sequence is generally cereal, fruits, vegetables, meat, egg yolk, fish and whole egg. As each new item is added, three to four days should lapse before another item is added.
467. **A.**—Food intolerance is not necessarily associated with fever or drowsiness.
468. **C.**—Sweet potatoes and squash are high flatus producers; pepper and onions are irritating substances, thus they should be withheld until the child has developed a full repertory of foods.
469. **D.**—The dietary regimen should be developed in conjunction with the child and his parents within the framework of the child's dietary history. Caloric intake should be cut down while maintaining adequate nutritional needs for proteins, carbohydrates, fats, vitamins and minerals.
470. **B.**—It is very important to bring about weight loss gradually. A pound of body fat represents an excess intake of 3500 calories.
471. **D.**—The person must decrease caloric intake by 1000 calories per day.
472. **C.**—An unexpected vacation as a factor influencing obesity can easily be corrected since it is not ingrained in the individual's developmental environment.
473. **B.**—An egg a day or at least 3 to 5 a week is a good practice to follow.
474. **C.**—Milk is our main source of calcium in foods. It also contributes fine quality proteins, vitamins, and many other nutrients.
475. **A.**—Spaghetti is an excellent source of carbohydrates.
476. **D.**—Carrots are high in Vitamin A.
477. **B.**—Poultry could be substituted with peas, nuts, or peanut butter.
478. **D.**—Spinach is an excellent source of Vitamin A.
479. **B.**—Fish belong to the protein-containing basic group.
480. **A.**—Bread and cereals may be used at least four times daily.
481. **C.**—Dried fruits are rich in iron.
482. **B.**—Peanut butter is a good substitute for meat, fish, poultry, or eggs.
483. **B.**—Strawberries are rich in Vitamin C.
484. **A.**—Broccoli and all "greens" are high in Vitamin A.
485. **C.**—In calcium content, ½ cup ice cream is equal to ¼ glass of milk.
486. **D.**—Liver is an important source of iron and Vitamin B.
487. **D.**—Raisins, being dried fruits, are rich in iron.
488. **A.**—Spinach is a rich source of Vitamin A.
489. **C.**—In calcium content, ½ cup creamed cottage cheese is equal to ½ glass of milk.
490. **B.**—Two medium tomatoes are equal in Vitamin C content to 2 cups of juice.
491. **A.**—Cantaloupe is a valuable source of Vitamin A.
492. **D.**—Dried fruits such as prunes are valuable for iron.
493. **D.**—Growth spurts would be associated with increased appetite to meet the biological demands of the increasing activity level of the growing child.
494. **C.**—Overfeeding, rather than underfeeding is likely to cause colic.
495. **B.**—Because of the child's slower rate of growth following the first year of life, his need for food is correspondingly decreased. This is normal and should never be a signal for the mother to force a child to eat or to become anxious lest he starve.
496. **A.**—The infant should be given foods that are easy for him to hold and feed to himself. This will be both a pleasurable experience and the first step toward self-feeding.
497. **C.**—If the mother's milk is diminishing in quantity or if she has to return to work outside the home, the infant may be weaned before 6 months of age.
498. **D.**—The infant is already under a physical and emotional strain from his illness.

499. **A.**—Eating too much between meals would otherwise have an adverse affect on a child's appetite for regular meals.
500. **C.**—Children should not be coaxed, bribed, or forced to eat. The child identifies with his family and enjoys eating with them and joining in the conversation. Mealtime is a good time for parents to answer questions, provided this does not distract the child from eating.
501. **D.**—Each child has definite likes and dislikes. Children generally like plain food served attractively in separate dishes.
502. **B.**—The need for vitamin D can be met by exposure of the skin to sunlight.
503. **A.**—The normal relatively slow weight gain with less need for food from 1 to 5 years of age can be readily misinterpreted by anxious parents as anorexia.
504. **C.**—Organic diseases such as anemia and tuberculosis are inherently associated with anorexia.
505. **D.**—Otherwise known as vitamin B_6, it is essential for hemoglobin, serotonin, and histamine formation.
506. **A.**—Kwashiorkor, on the other hand, is a protein deficiency syndrome.
507. **C.**—Loose, wrinkled skin is characteristic of marasmus resulting from loss of fat layers. A child suffering from kwashiorkor may not unduly lose fat layers.
508. **B.**—Iodine is essential for thyroxin production.
509. **B.**—Consideration should be primarily geared to the cultural aspects of food acceptance by children of various ethnic and racial backgrounds.
510. **C.**—Health education is always a supplement to, never a substitute for, interviewing and conference routines.
511. **D.**—Planning is indeed the essence behind any successful health education program. Above all, it should be dynamic. It should be tried in different ways. Curriculum development is not at all crucial in parents' group discussions.
512. **D.**—Research in education has demonstrated again and again that people learn better when they experience something through more than one of their senses, or when things are presented in more than one way at the same time. Although very expensive, films are often an excellent teaching device. Film strips are much less attractive than films, but are much cheaper and often provide a good take-off for discussion.
513. **B.**—The nurse is in a strategic spot to prevent tension before it arises, before it is even in the potential stage.
514. **C.**—The mother should not be nursing the baby the very first time the older child sees him since it is likely to cause the child to feel neglected.
515. **D.**—A certain amount of regression can be expected in a situation like this. Assure the mother that many other children would feel the same way as her child does. The child must be made to feel he is not being displaced.
516. **B.**—A baby's needs should be met as promptly as possible but promptly does not necessarily mean instantly.
517. **A.**—The notion that parents only serve, never guide, is one of the unfortunate distortions of the self-demand idea. The idea behind "flexible schedule" is virtually the same as the idea behind "permissiveness with limits," and there is much a mother can do to establish a flexible, orderly routine.
518. **D.**—Most two-year-old children are beginning to feel the need for companionship, and the day care center could be an excellent place for them when the mother or significant other cannot be with them.
519. **C.**—The presence of a good mother substitute would minimize, if not prevent, the impact of separation anxiety.
520. **C.**—Availability of pots, pans, bowls and boxes would encourage the child to put in and take out things to his heart's content.
521. **D.**—It should be made clear to parents that social behavior has its developmental phase too.
522. **A.**—It is necessary to reassure parents that shoes are not necessary for support in the average child.
523. **C.**—Other children do not have to miss

school as long as they remain well. Antiseptic lotion is not necessary; the child, however, should be kept from scratching the lesions. Application of an antipruritic lotion to the lesions, such as calamine lotion, may alleviate itching. Chickenpox can be spread to others through droplet infection and by direct or indirect contact, hence, the necessity for isolating the patient.

524. **D.**—Toilet training should be started when the toddler is physiologically and psychologically ready. The family environment should be relaxed as well.

525. **C.**—It is very important to utilize the parents' own resources for any program involving children and families.

526. **C.**—The affected persons are principally males in sex-linked recessive inheritance patterns.

527. **A.**—Cleft palate may be due to an autosomal dominant gene.

528. **B.**—Poor diagnostic procedures would likely miss a number of congenital defects, hence be associated with corresponding low statistical count.

529. **C.**—Congenital malformations could hardly be pinpointed to any one cause. They are the result of the interaction between genetic and environmental factors.

530. **B.**—The sons of an affected male are normal, the daughters carriers.

531. **D.**—Klinefelter's syndrome is one of the more common chromosomal disorders and is the result of random errors of meiosis. Recurrence risks are generally not increased.

532. **D.**—No nurse is ever expected to prescribe an antibiotic for any patient.

533. **B.**—Rheumatic fever is commonly seen in the school age group.

534. **D.**—Acne should be treated as early as possible. Medical attention should be readily sought since acne can produce permanent scars.

535. **C.**—The permanent color of the iris will be manifested in 50% of children by 6 months of age and in all children by 12 months.

536. **A.**—The risk that a carrier will marry another carrier is high if he marries a close relative.

537. **A.**—Stretching the iliolumbar ligament to prevent structural scoliosis has been recommended. This is done by lateral bending to the opposite side while the pelvis is stabilized.

538. **D.**—In the severely involved or nonambulatory patient, positioning devices must be used most of the time.

539. **A.**—Chromosomes are the threadlike structures which carry the genes; they are composed of nucleic acid and protein.

540. **C.**—Some evidence indicates that genes are actually segments of DNA and that possibly thousands of genes exist in each molecule.

541. **B.**—Alleles are alternate forms of a gene.

542. **B.**—If both parents are carriers, two children will be heterozygous normal; one child will be homozygous abnormal; and one will be homozygous normal.

543. **C.**—The principal organ systems of the body are developing during the first trimester of pregnancy, hence the importance of protecting the woman during this period from infections such as rubella and toxoplasmosis which may cause congenital anomalies.

544. **C.**—Hereditary diseases and a predisposition to certain other diseases are fixed at time of conception, while congenital diseases can occur at any time.

CHAPTER IV

Developmental Problems and Nursing Care

INTRODUCTION

As people are born, grow, and live, they also die. Health deviations can occur anytime in one's life span from conception through death. Developmental problems commonly take place during the conceptual and gestational periods, although their clinical manifestations have the greatest impact during infancy and childhood. To learn that their infant is born abnormal is a great shock to a family. This situation bears important implications for the total development of the child, the nature of the parent-and-child relations, the delivery of health care, and the overall health status of the society in which they live. A sympathetic, tactful, knowledgeable, and clinically competent nurse can do a great deal to alleviate some of the distress that the problem brings. She can help the child and his family actualize their potentials and utilize their resources for a healthful life.

The content of this chapter is largely presented in situation form to enable you to analyze a complex situation and examine the relationship of its component parts, evaluate your ability to understand the significance of various clinical observations, recognize basic principles underlying specific modes of intervention, and speculate on the probable effects of specific nursing actions. Items are also included to test your ability to recall previously learned facts and ideas.

A. Diarrhea

Directions: This part of the test consists of a situation followed by a series of incomplete statements. Study the situation and select the best answer to each statement that follows.

Situation: Jed Graham, a 5-month-old boy, was brought to the hospital by his mother for loose bowel movement and fever of two days' duration. He weighed 11.5 pounds. His anterior fontanel was sunken and his skin turgor poor. He had four watery and foul-smelling stools in the last two hours. Jed was admitted immediately with a diagnosis of diarrhea of unknown origin.

1. A blood specimen was drawn from his jugular vein on admission. Jed was restrained by using a (an)
   A. elbow restraint
   B. abdominal restraint
   C. mummy restraint
   D. clove hitch restraint   (13:342)

2. During the procedure, the nurse was basically responsible for
   A. interviewing mother
   B. positioning infant properly
   C. observing sterility
   D. preparing parenteral solution (13:342)

Developmental Problems

3. Intravenous therapy was started. The most important responsibility of the nurse was to
   A. flush tube as soon as solution stops dripping
   B. remove needle as soon as bottle gets empty
   C. add new bottle of solution when present one is empty, with or without doctor's orders
   D. frequently check flow of solution and regulate flow as ordered (13:343)

4. What is the observation that would be the earliest sign of circulatory overload?
   A. puffy eyelids
   B. high pitched cry
   C. oliguria
   D. increased respirations (13:342)

5. Which of the following is *not a* safety measure to minimize the possibility of circulatory overload?
   A. speed up IV rate as soon as you get behind
   B. use of Soluset with 100 cc chamber
   C. use of small quantity bottles (250 cc or 500 cc)
   D. observing urine output hourly (13:342)

6. If 150 cc of 5% Dextrose solution is to be consumed in 8 hours, to how many microdrops per minute should you regulate the flow?
   A. 15
   B. 19
   C. 25
   D. 29 (13:343)

7. What amount of urine output is evidence of good renal function for Jed?
   A. 600–700 cc/24 hrs
   B. 400–500 cc/24 hrs
   C. 100–300 cc/24 hrs
   D. 30–60 cc/24 hrs (28:134)

8. If diarrhea persists, Jed will develop acidosis because of an increased loss of
   A. calcium and chlorides
   B. sodium and potassium
   C. sodium and sulfates
   D. bicarbonates and phosphates (13:338)

9. Which of the following signs of dehydration would Jed exhibit?
   A. fever, anuria, slow pulse, edema
   B. poor skin turgor, weight loss, bulging fontanel
   C. pallor, perio-orbital edema, fever, rapid pulse
   D. sunken fontanel, poor skin turgor, oliguria (13:336)

10. In charting Jed's stool, the nurse should note the following, *except*
    A. color, size
    B. odor, consistency
    C. presence of blood or pus
    D. character of stool passed at home (13:446)

11. Jed's temperature was always taken by axilla. The primary reason for this was to
    A. prevent undue stimulation of intestines
    B. minimize Jed's discomfort
    C. prevent cross infection
    D. abide by hospital policy (13:346)

12. Strict isolation was enforced on Jed, and proper isolation technique was subsequently observed. The specific isolation measures included the following, *except*
    A. using disposable diapers
    B. wearing of gown by all persons coming in contact with Jed
    C. keeping mother from direct contact with Jed
    D. boiling bottles and nipples after use (13:346)

13. If Jed's temperature gets subnormal, the nurse should
    A. report sign promptly to doctor
    B. place additional blankets over him
    C. give him tepid sponge bath
    D. place him in incubator (13:346)

14. If a hot water bottle is applied, the nurse should *first*
    A. take Jed's temperature
    B. refer procedure to nurse in charge

C. get mother's consent
D. examine bottle for leaks (13:346)

15. Oral fluids were ordered as soon as Jed's diarrhea was checked. Important guidelines to be observed in feeding Jed included the following *except*
    A. forcing fluids — leads to vomiting
    B. small, frequent feedings
    C. checking physician's order before giving formula
    D. adding solid foods gradually (13:345)

Directions: For each of the following multiple choice questions, select the ONE most appropriate answer.

16. The acid-base balance of the body is maintained by the concentration of what *element* in the body?
    A. oxygen
    B. hydrogen   ↑ ions — acid
    C. calcium   ↓ — alkalosis
    D. potassium   (27:27)

17. An increased loss of sodium and potassium from the extracellular fluid would result in
    A. alkalosis
    B. acidosis
    C. osmolar dehydration
    D. hypermolar dehydration (27:27)

18. The main components in fluid-electrolyte homeostasis are
    A. solutes and solvents
    B. cations and anions
    C. intracellular and extracellular fluids
    D. none of the above (27:27)

19. The most important cation of the intracellular fluid is
    A. phosphate
    B. calcium
    C. potassium
    D. chloride (27:27)

20. The most important cation and anion of the entracellular fluid are respectively
    A. potassium and sodium
    B. sodium and chloride
    C. calcium and chloride
    D. sodium and phosphate (27:27)

21. Unchecked diarrhea is very dangerous because it can readily lead to
    A. metabolic alkalosis
    B. metabolic acidosis
    C. fluid-electrolyte imbalance
    D. osmolaric dehydration (27:26)

22. Increased extracellular fluid in infancy is extremely important because of the following facts, *except*
    A. infant's body surface is approximately three times that of adult in proportion to body fluid volume
    B. infant's metabolic rate is higher than that of the adult
    C. extracellular fluid is approximately one-half of the infant's body weight
    D. infant rapidly depletes his fluid volume (27:28)

23. Which of the statements below is *not* true of "water intoxication"?
    A. it occurs when extra intracellular fluid is replaced too rapidly
    B. the extracellular fluids become hypotonic and the intracellular fluid becomes hypertonic
    C. it is a response to over-saturation of the child's body
    D. the condition is frequently associated with signs of cerebral edema (27:29)

24. Isolation of a child with diarrhea implies that
    A. all who come in contact with the child observe isolation routine
    B. visitors will be limited to parents only
    C. toys given to child need not be limited
    D. A and B (27:30)

25. When the child's diarrhea has been adequately controlled, the child's oral intake will be reinstituted. Specific guidelines include the following, *except*
    A. introducing oral intake in graduated steps of increasing volume and solid content

Developmental Problems 113

B. encouraging child to take fluids and solids as tolerated and desired
C. observing accurately and reporting child's tolerance to changing oral intake
D. seeing to it that child receives proper volume of fluids at specified times
(27:30)

B. Vomiting

Directions: **This part of the test consists of a situation followed by a series of incomplete statements. Study the situation and select the best answer to complete each statement that follows.**

Situation: Billy Ball, a 1-month-old infant, was admitted with a possible diagnosis of pyloric stenosis. His mother reports that he is always hungry.

26. Knowing about the pathophysiology, what symptom(s) would you look for when caring for Billy?
    A. projectile vomiting following meals
    B. dehydration and decrease in stools
    C. sudden recurring pain
    D. A and B (13:349)

27. Frequently there is an acid-base imbalance with this condition. Which of the following would *most* likely be found clinically?
    A. change in pH from 7.3 to 7.0
    B. increased pCO_2 ↓ pH = ↓ serum cl
    C. change in pH from 7.3 to 7.5
    D. B and C (13:350)

28. Feeding Billy entails paying attention to many details. Which of the following would be the *least* important detail to follow?
    A. observing for signs of a pyloric wave which indicates increased activity
    B. thickening the formula to prevent vomiting and slow digestion
    C. administering anticholinergic medication (belladonna) 30 minutes before feeding
    D. burping frequently to prevent build-up of air in stomach (13:350,351)

29. You notice that when Billy sleeps on his back, his head turns to one side with his arm extending on this same side and his opposite arm flexed. Which of the following *best* describes this position? It is
    A. called the tonic neck reflex and is normal for this age group
    B. a Moro reflex and indicates that Billy has regressed somewhat
    C. a coincidence that he is lying this way. It means nothing.
    D. not unusual for infants to adopt a particular position during sleep (13:286)

30. A day or two after the operation you are interested in increasing sensory input for Billy. You might *best* accomplish this with
    A. mobiles across the crib
    B. wind-up musical instruments
    C. bright colors and patterns on crib
    D. bodily contact and voice tone (13:282)

31. Which of the following would best help minimize vomiting in infants?
    A. feed infant first, then bathe
    B. place on right side in elevated position
    C. place on left side, slightly elevated
    D. feed more frequently (13:350)

32. In case of vomiting, to prevent Billy from aspirating vomitus, the nurse could do any of the following measures, *except*
    A. turn his head to side
    B. place him on his right side
    C. place him flat on his back
    D. place him on his abdomen, his head turned (13:348)

33. Important considerations in the nursing care of Billy should include the following, *except*
    A. charting whenever he voids, noting exact time and estimating amount of urine voided
    B. making friends with him
    C. giving treatments just before feeding time
    D. giving special attention to skin care, particularly face, neck and behind ears (13:348)

34. The nurse understands that vomiting is different from <u>rumination</u> in that the latter indicates
    A. voluntary bringing up of small amounts of food from stomach shortly after feeding
    B. spitting up of formula in small amounts and drooling from infant's mouth
    C. increase in size of circular musculature of pylorus
    D. faulty feeding technique (13:347)

35. The most important consideration in the management of Billy is to check his vomiting since persistent vomiting can readily result in alkalosis. Which of the following may occur if alkalosis is severe?
    A. convulsion
    B. dehydration
    C. tetany
    D. A and C (13:346)

C. Cleft Lip and Palate

Situation: Michael Stewart, age 1 month, was born with a cleft lip and palate. He was admitted to the pediatric department and had plastic surgery for repair of the lip.

36. In the recovery room, Michael suddenly becomes cyanotic. Which would you do *first?*
    A. call for assistance
    B. administer oxygen
    C. suction the nasopharynx
    D. insert an oral airway (13:229)

37. Which of the following are important in Michael's postoperative nursing care?
    1. feeding him with a rubber-tipped syringe
    2. removing his elbow restraints while he is sleeping
    3. following his feeding with water to help cleanse the suture line
    4. cleaning the suture line with hydrogen peroxide after feedings
    5. placing him on his abdomen after his feeding
    A. 1, 2, and 3
    B. 1, 2, and 4
    C. 2, 3, and 5
    D. 2, 4, and 5 (13:229)

38. After nausea and vomiting cease, fluids should <u>not be given</u> to Michael
    A. with cup or side of spoon
    B. with straw, nipple or syringe
    C. inside of mouth
    D. in center of mouth (13:229)

39. The best immediate postoperative position, when Michael is conscious, is
    A. on abdomen with head turned to one side
    B. on side
    C. on back with head turned to side
    D. flat (13:229)

40. Which of the following statements are applicable to cleft palate anomaly?
    A. the exact cause is unknown
    B. surgery is discouraged until about 4 years of age if speech defects are present
    C. it involves only the soft palate
    D. it involves only the hard palate (13:228)

41. Complications related to cleft palate are which of the following?
    A. loss of hearing, dental decay
    B. dental decay, frequent upper respiratory infections
    C. stridor
    D. sluggish choke reflex (13:230)

Situation: Jimmy Jones, who has a unilateral cleft lip, was admitted to the pediatric unit from the newborn nursery.

42. His mother and father are distraught over this obvious defect. The nurse's best response in supporting the family would be to
    A. place Jimmy in a crib where other children and parents could not see him
    B. state that Jimmy's deformity is mild in comparison with others she had seen
    C. agree with the parents that the deformity is difficult for them to accept

Developmental Problems 115

(D.) treat Jimmy as a normal infant and at the same time allow the parents to voice their feelings of disappointment (13:225)

43. Jimmy's parents were concerned about the surgery to be performed for repair of the cleft lip. Which of the following would *not* be an appropriate nursing measure related to their instruction?
   A. tell them not to worry about that now, as surgery will not be done until Jimmy is 5 years old
   B. show them "before and after" photographs of infants who have undergone repair
   C. arrange for the surgeon to discuss with the parents the procedure to be done
   D. introduction of postoperative measures which the mother can learn (13:225)

44. Which of the following is a true statement about postoperative nursing care following cleft lip repair?
   A. a hard nipple is used in all cases because the repair increases the power of the child's suck
   B. the child's mother should not be allowed to give him any care because the suture line is too fragile
   C. though restraints are necessary, he should be given opportunity to exercise his arms
   D. he should be positioned on his abdomen (13:225)

45. Which of the following is *not* affected by cleft palate deformities?
   A. swallowing
   B. breathing
   C. speech
   D. neck mobility (13:225)

46. Which of the following are nursing priorities in the postoperative management of Jimmy?
   1. keeping the mouth clean and free of irritation
   2. maintenance of an open airway
   3. provision of scheduled milk feedings
   4. feeding the child with a straw
   5. meeting child's needs promptly to prevent crying
   A. 1, 2 and 5
   B. 2, 4 and 5
   C. 2, 3, 4 and 5
   D. 1, 2, 3 and 5 (13:229)

D. Meningomyelocele and Hydrocephalus

Situation: Sally Ann was admitted to the pediatric unit immediately after birth. A large bulging purplish mass located in the central area of the spine is noted. Diagnosis of meningomyelocele is made.

47. Which of the following clinical signs may be seen?
   A. flaccid paralysis of arms and legs, lack of bowel and bladder function
   B. flaccid paralysis of arms and legs, hydrocephalus
   C. flaccid paralysis of legs, absence of sensation in feet, clubbed feet
   D. flaccid paralysis of arms, lack of bowel function (13:245,246)

48. The nurse's *prime* concern in caring for Sally Ann is
   A. providing O_2 because of infant's labored respirations
   B. keeping the deformity covered when parents visit
   C. passive exercise of arms and legs
   D. prevention of infection of sac (13:246)

49. Which of the following groups of symptoms might be seen if hydrocephalus (noncommunicating) were present?
   A. increase in head size, constricted scalp veins, high-pitched cry, vomiting
   B. increase in head size, irritability, vomiting, dilated scalp veins
   C. irritability, decreased head size, vomiting, constricted scalp veins
   D. low-pitched, grunting cry, increased head size, vomiting (13:252)

Sally Ann is now one month old. During the past month the tumor has increased in size and the wall is thinner. Surgery is performed.

50. Postoperatively, her position is likely to be
    A. flat, on abdomen, turned side to side with care
    B. on Bradford frame, on abdomen, tilted with head slightly lower than body
    C. propped on side with operative side protected with dressing and brace
    D. on back with operative area over the opening of the Bradford frame
    (13:248)

51. Following the operation, you would expect Sally Ann to have
    A. only temporary dysfunction
    B. paralysis of legs, urinary and fecal incontinence
    C. rupture and ulcerative perforation
    D. no dysfunction due to surgery beyond immediate postoperative period
    (13:249)

52. In caring for Sally Ann a week postoperatively you should
    1. change position from side to side every two hours
    2. pick her up for her evaporated milk feedings
    3. measure her head daily
    4. crede her bladder to empty it
    5. give her an enema every other day
       A. 1, 2 and 3
       B. 1, 2 and 4
       C. 2, 3, and 5
       D. 3, 4, and 5
    (13:249)

53. Rehabilitation programs for children following repair of myelomeningocele should include
    1. a bowel and bladder training program
    2. a feeding program
    3. speech therapy
    4. braces and physiotherapy
       A. 1 and 3
       B. 1 and 4
       C. 2 and 3
       D. 3 and 4
    (13:250)

54. Sally Ann developed hydrocephalus. A shunt was performed. Postoperatively, the nurse's decision to change her position frequently is based on several reasons. Which of the following would *not* apply?
    A. because of the weight of her head, Sally Ann cannot lift her head to turn it to relieve pressure to areas of skin on her head and body
    B. because she cannot easily move about, she will be predisposed to hypostatic pneumonia
    C. to increase Sally Ann's visual and auditory sensory input
    D. to promote flow of cerebrospinal fluid around occluded area
    (13:254)

E. Cystic Fibrosis

Situation: Susan Lim, 3 years old and the youngest of four children, has been admitted to the hospital with a history of poor weight gain and repeated upper respiratory infections. In talking with the mother you learn that Susan had bronchopneumonia at 18 months of age and has recently had large, foul smelling, bulky stools. The doctor has made the diagnosis of cystic fibrosis.

55. Which of the following pathophysiological findings is *not* present in cystic fibrosis?
    A. excessive secretion of the exocrine glands of the body
    B. obstruction of air passages in the lungs
    C. inability to metabolize certain amino acids
    D. production of excessive amounts of sodium and chloride in the sweat
    (13:375)

56. Medications which may be given to Susan include all of the following *except*
    A. pancreatic substitutes
    B. fat soluble vitamins
    C. salt tablets during hot weather
    D. antibiotics
    (13:375)

Developmental Problems

57. Susan is to have ⅛% Neosynephrine by aerosol and postural drainage at home. Her mother asks you when to administer the aerosol treatments. You should tell her to give it
   1. half an hour after her postural drainage
   2. just before her postural drainage
   3. immediately after meals
   4. half an hour before meals
   A. 1 and 3
   B. 1 and 4
   C. 2 and 3
   D. 2 and 4 (13:376-77)

58. Cystic fibrosis is a congenital disease inherited as an autosomal trait. According to the Mendelian Law the following phenomena would be demonstrated in Susan's family history, *except*
   A. her parents must be carriers
   B. each child in family has a one in four chance of having disease
   C. no child in family will be normal
   D. two siblings will be heterozygous normal (13:373)

59. Usually, only a trypsin test is made to establish the diagnosis of cystic fibrosis. What kind of specimen is being used to test for tryptic activity?
   A. stool
   B. urine
   C. sweat
   D. blood (13:374)

60. What type of diet would be indicated for Susan?
   A. high caloric, high protein, low fat
   B. low caloric, high protein, low fat
   C. high caloric, low protein, high fat
   D. high carbohydrate, high protein, low fat (13:375)

61. Caring for Susan during hospitalization should be primarily geared towards
   A. providing her physical care and emotional support
   B. teaching mother routines of such care at home
   C. helping family adjust to new life style imposed by Susan's special needs
   D. all of the above (13:376)

62. This is the first time that Susan is to receive intermittent positive pressure treatments. After obtaining the necessary equipment and medication, the *first* thing you should do to lessen Susan's fears would be to
   A. turn on the oxygen before starting the treatment
   B. position her in bed
   C. explain the entire procedure to her
   D. let her hold the mouthpiece and tubing (13:377)

63. Which of the following would best describe Susan if she were a healthy three-year-old?
   A. grows rapidly, feeds self, names figures in a picture
   B. helps dress herself, attempts to sing songs, talks in complete sentences
   C. sits quietly at the table, has a vocabulary of approximately 900 words, goes on errands outside the home
   D. is toilet trained at night, understands time, participates in imaginative play (13:532)

64. Considering Susan's developmental and therapeutic needs, which of the following play activities would be *most* desirable?
   A. cutting out paper dolls
   B. jumping rope with her friends
   C. playing with windmills
   D. stringing large beads (13:531)

65. During the terminal stage of cystic fibrosis the child is in respiratory distress and has frequent episodes of coughing. The nurse caring for her should do all of the following, *except*
   A. plan her nursing care so as to conserve her energy
   B. place her in a croupette with oxygen and moisture to help liquefy secretions
   C. give her cough medicine, such as codeine and terpin hydrate
   D. support her while coughing (13:376,377,378)

F. Diabetes Mellitus

Directions: For each of the following multiple choice questions, select the ONE most appropriate answer.

66. Diabetes in children differs from diabetes in adults in which of the following ways?
    1. the onset is slower
    2. the condition is seldom managed without insulin
    3. the psychological implications tend to be greater
    4. the preadolescent is easier to regulate
    A. 1 and 2
    B. 1 and 4
    C. 2 and 3
    D. all of the above (13:655,656)

67. Which of the following situations does *not* increase insulin requirements in a diabetic child?
    A. acute infection
    B. emotional disturbance
    C. surgical operation
    D. strenuous exercise (13:656)

68. Diabetes in children can be controlled by
    A. diet alone
    B. diet and oral hypoglycemic agents
    C. diet and insulin
    D. insulin alone (13:658)

69. An adolescent with diabetes tells the nurse that she's been asked to join the co-ed swimming team. "Do you think Dr. M. will agree to my swimming; I'm a good swimmer." What is the best response to her question?
    A. "Probably not, because of your unstable condition, but ask him."
    B. "Work on getting your diabetes under control and then ask him."
    C. "You must be thrilled, ask him today. He might say 'yes,' if you agree to be careful."
    D. "I'm certain he will be interested, but don't be disappointed if he says 'no.'"

70. If a diabetic patient, whose skin and mouth are dry, complains of thirst, you are alerted to the possibility of
    A. insulin shock
    B. diabetic acidosis
    C. ketosis
    D. renal failure (13:655)

71. Manifestations of insulin shock which a child might show are
    1. diarrhea
    2. dilated pupils
    3. behavioral changes
    4. rapid pulse
    5. abdominal pain
    A. 1, 2 and 3
    B. 1, 3 and 5
    C. 2, 3 and 4
    D. 2, 4 and 5 (13:658)

72. Which of the following is *not* a sign of diabetic acidosis?
    A. hyperglycemia
    B. elevated plasma carbon dioxide content
    C. shift in blood pH toward 7.30
    D. depletion of glycogen stores in the liver (13:658)

73. A 12-year-old diabetic could be expected to do which of the following, assuming he has had adequate instruction?
    A. keep records, draw up and give insulin to himself, help to plan his diet
    B. test urine, keep records, draw up but not administer the insulin
    C. test urine, keep records, draw up insulin but have it checked by an adult
    D. test urine, draw up and administer the insulin, but have an adult plan his diet (13:659)

74. If a diabetic child tells you, "something is wrong, I don't feel good," your immediate response is to
    A. sit down with him for incidental counseling
    B. give him sugar or fruit juice or a candy bar
    C. contact his parents for further information
    D. refer him to a medical doctor (13:658)

75. If strict diet management is prescribed for a child with diabetes, the goal is to

Developmental Problems

    A. have the child develop self-control
    B. prevent insulin shock
    C. keep urine aglycosuric
    D. test urine for sugar and give insulin if needed   (13:656)

76. Which of the following is an indication of diabetes common in children and *not in adults*?
    A. bedwetting — Polyuria
    B. thumbsucking
    C. weight gain
    D. increased thirst   (13:654)

Directions: This part of the test consists of a situation followed by a series of incomplete statements. Study the situation and select the best answer to complete each statement that follows.

Situation: Mrs. S. and 15-year-old Debby are visiting the clinic. Debby has had diabetes since she was 11 years old. She is now experiencing problems with managing her diabetes. When Debby leaves the room, her mother expresses concern about Debby's behavior.

77. Mrs. S. tells you, "Debby has always taken pride in managing her own diet, but since she's started high school she's not sticking to her diet. What can I do?" Your *best* answer should be
    A. her body requires more food right now, Debby needs the food she is eating
    B. Debby has a need to be like her peers; be patient and reencourage her
    C. Debby can get into real difficulties; talk with her teacher and the school nurse
    D. I'll work with Debby to write out a diet for her to follow during this period of adjustment   (13:660)

78. Mrs. S. tells you that she is happy that Debby is taking an interest in religion. You recognize this as
    A. normal for this age group — sense of identity
    B. an expression of fear on Debby's part
    C. a sign of guilt from Debby
    D. B and C   (13:682)

79. Mrs. S. tells you, "Debby is so emotional lately; she cries about so many things. Is this reaction due to her unstable diabetic condition?" Your *best* response would be
    A. yes, as the diabetic condition stabilizes, so will Debby's emotional state
    B. teen-agers are normally emotional, but Debby's anxiety about her condition may add to this instability
    C. this is normal for teen-agers; she will outgrow it as she matures
    D. there is no relationship between Debby's diabetic condition and her crying episodes   (13:660)

80. Freud might interpret Debby's concern for eating to allay her fears as
    A. emergence of the superego
    B. an expression of denial
    C. the id surfacing
    D. B and C   (13:656,658)

81. Of the following, which phase(s) would you associate with the adolescent?
    A. reflective thinking
    B. romantic infatuation
    C. symbolism
    D. A and B   (13:680)

G. Autism

Situation: Tommy Smith is a three-year old whose behavior since birth has caused his parents concern. Originally he was diagnosed as having unknown brain damage at birth resulting in mental retardation. However, at the children's diagnostic and evaluation center he was seen by a psychologist who established the diagnosis of autism.

82. The following behavior could be expected of Tommy, *except*
    A. strumming of his lips
    B. banging his head
    C. refusing to communicate verbally
    D. clinging to his mother   (13:593,594)

83. A part of the regimen provided for Tommy should include the following, *except*
    A. reinforcing positive behavior with candy
    B. reinforcing fantasy world which child sees

C. good, physical care
D. play therapy (13:594)

84. Autism could easily be confused with childhood schizophrenia. Which of the following behaviors is *not* directly related to schizophrenia?
    A. tactile and visual hallucinations
    B. inability to discern body boundaries
    C. inappropriate affect
    D. strong, intense bonds with one person perceived to be necessary for existence (15:100)

85. Which of the following is a true statement about the cause of schizophrenia?
    A. heredity is a causative factor in all cases of schizophrenia
    B. family dynamics have not been seen as a causative factor as the schizophrenia is felt to be isolated to the individual only
    C. several theories are being researched but no one cause has been proved
    D. biochemical defects have not been seen in any schizophrenics (30:33,34,35)

Directions: For each of the following multiple choice questions, select the ONE most appropriate answer.

86. The first person to describe autistic children as a special group and consequently incited a growing interest in this problem was
    A. Freud
    B. Itard
    C. Pinel
    D. Kanner (30:7)

87. Which of the statements below is *not* generally true about autism?
    A. boys are affected more often than girls
    B. parents of autistic children are likely to be of higher intelligence and educational level than average
    C. autistic babies scream a great deal especially on waking from sleep and cannot be comforted or soothed unless subjected to continuous motion
    D. autism is a condition that occurs as often as total deafness and more often than total blindness (30:11,13)

88. Which of the following ages represents the span when autistic behavior is most obvious?
    A. 1–7
    B. 2–5
    C. 6–9
    D. 7–13 (30:13)

89. Which of the senses would be *least* sensitive in Tommy?
    A. sight
    B. hearing
    C. smell
    D. touch (30:12,13)

90. The most common reason why autistic children are often confused with words that usually occur in pairs, e.g., "brush" may be called "comb" or "sock" may be called "shoe" is that they
    A. do not know the difference
    B. cannot learn the difference
    C. cannot call the proper word to mind quickly
    D. have very little appreciation for anything in their surroundings (30:17)

91. Which of the following behaviors is *least* characteristic of autistic children?
    A. confusing two words that are opposite in meaning
    B. muddling the order of letters inside words
    C. repeating words or phrases heard in the past which may have little or no meaning for the child
    D. muddling the order of words inside sentences (30:15,17)

Directions: The following items refer to categories of behavior and their corresponding manifestations as commonly observed in autistic children. Match the following numbered items with the most appropriate lettered items.

92. Aloofness and social withdrawal (30:24)
93. Resistance to change (30:25)
94. Socially embarrassing behavior (30:27)
95. Clumsiness in skilled movements (30:23)

A. Routinely tap on chair before sitting down, turning around three times in the course of a meal

B. Point down instead of up, and move the left arm instead of the right and so on
C. Does not listen if you speak to him, shows no interest or sympathy if you are in pain or distress
D. Never tell lies

Directions: For each of the following multiple choice questions, select the ONE most appropriate answer.

96. Some autistic children remain difficult, but the majority do improve at least to some extent after the first few years. The biggest change is usually seen in what aspect?
    A. motor
    B. social and emotional
    C. cognitive
    D. language (30:112,113)

97. An educational program that would seem best suited for autistic children is which one of the following?
    A. open classroom
    B. social and emotional
    C. Montessori
    D. psychotherapeutic (30:55)

98. Which of the following is *least* accepted as a reason underlying the belief that autism is due to emotional causes?
    A. it has been shown that orphanages or institutions which give no "mothering" to their babies, produce autistic children
    B. most autistic children, when they are young, have many behavior problems, especially in relating to other people and in showing affection
    C. various writers have reported that parents of autistic children had abnormal personalities
    D. in most cases, siblings of an autistic child are healthy and normal (30:34)

99. Which of the following would be *least* effective in the management of an autistic child if he goes into temper tantrums?
    A. never give things the child wants while he is actually in tantrums
    B. ignore the child while he is screaming but as soon as tantrum stops he should be given lots of attention, praise, and some other suitable reward
    C. ignore the child without eventual reward
    D. slap the child when something has to be done in a hurry (30:34)

100. Which of the following principles is *least* helpful when teaching autistic children?
    A. children are likely to learn behavior which is rewarded and are likely to refrain from behavior which has unpleasant results
    B. new skills are learned more easily if they are initially presented as a whole rather than broken down into very tiny simple steps
    C. children can be encouraged to try new skills by prompting them, fairly obviously at first, then less and less as time goes on
    D. link new learning with skills which are already familiar and which give pleasure (30:85,89)

101. Autistic children, once they have become reasonably cooperative and willing to learn, can be taught many simple tasks. Which of the following tasks is best to start an autistic child with?
    A. clearing leaves from the garden
    B. putting out the milk bottle
    C. pushing a trolley in a supermarket
    D. laying the table with cutlery (30:99)

102. Many autistic children enjoy traveling, once special fears of buses, cars or trains have been overcome. Which of the following guidelines would be *least* helpful when preparing this type of child for a vacation?
    A. be consistent and firm in social training
    B. take his favorite toys and clothes with you
    C. tell the child about the vacation just before taking off
    D. increase the scope of the vacation gradually (30:118)

103. Which of the following statements is *not* generally true about autistic children?

A. most autistic adolescents do not have the feeling of rebellion against their parents which is seen in normal young people
B. puberty is usually not delayed in autistic children, even though they often look younger than their actual age
C. menarche usually occurs within the same age range as with normal girls
D. autistic adolescents are usually as curious as their normal counterparts concerning conception and birth (30:6)

H. Syndromes of Cerebral Dysfunction

Cerebral Palsy

Directions: For each of the following multiple choice questions, select the ONE most appropriate answer.

104. Which of the following is the most frequent cause of permanent physical handicap among children?
 A. accidents
 B. infections
 C. cerebral palsy
 D. child abuse (22:10)

105. Which of the following fits the definition of cerebral palsy?
 A. it is a disorder of movement and posture due to a defect or lesion of the immature brain
 B. it comprises motor and other symptom complexes
 C. brain lesion or lesions are not progressive
 D. all of the above (22:10)

106. The leading diagnostic sign of cerebral palsy is
 A. motor function disorder
 B. encephalopathy
 C. seizure disorder at birth
 D. hydrocephalus (22:10)

107. Which of the following factors may play a role in the etiology of cerebral palsy?
 A. intra-uterine infections, anoxia, maternal metabolic disease, iso-immunization of the newborn
 B. prematurity, birth injury, infections, toxicosis, developmental anomaly of the brain
 C. both A and B
 D. neither A nor B (22:10,11)

108. Which of the following types of cerebral palsy comprise the largest group?
 A. ataxic
 B. atonic
 C. spastic
 D. athetoid (22:11,12)

109. A universal sign of spastic cerebral palsy is
 A. delay of motor milestone
 B. flexing of the arm and fisting of the hand in walking
 C. predominance of flexor posture
 D. spasticity of the hip abductors (22:12)

110. Hypotonia is marked and prolonged in what type of cerebral palsy?
 A. spastic
 B. atonic
 C. ataxic
 D. athetoid (22:14)

111. Athetoid cerebral palsy may be due to
 A. bilirubin encephalopathy
 B. intra-uterine infections
 C. both A and B
 D. neither A nor B (22:14)

112. Among the mixed type of cerebral palsy, which combination is most frequently encountered?
 A. athetosis and ataxia
 B. athetosis and spasticity
 C. spasticity and tremor ataxia
 D. ataxia and rigidity (22:14)

113. Which one of the following is *not* true about cerebral palsy?
 A. approximately one-third of such children score within normal range on intelligence tests
 B. associated nonmotor disabilities, such as mental retardation, are common
 C. about two-thirds of such children have some type of seizure disorder

Developmental Problems

D. likelihood of an intellectual deficit is greater when neuromuscular disability is severe (22:15)

114. Deafness and hearing loss are most often found in what type of cerebral palsy?
A. spastic
B. athetoid
C. atonic
D. rigid (22:17)

115. Measures for successful rehabilitation of a child with cerebral palsy should include the following, *except*
A. developmental training
B. physical therapy and orthopedic surgical procedures
C. combination of home program with formal therapy at treatment center
D. regular drug therapy (22:19)

116. Families of children with cerebral palsy need supportive counseling. Initially, counseling is directed toward
1. understanding implication of diagnosis
2. practical management of cerebral palsy child
3. handling feelings about having handicapped child
4. prospective treatment, hospitalization and surgical procedures
A. 1 and 3
B. 2 and 4
C. 1, 3 and 4
D. all of the above (22:22)

Directions: The following items refer to some etiological factors and the corresponding types of cerebral palsy largely influenced by these factors. Match the following numbered items with the ONE most appropriate lettered item.

117. Prematurity (22:35)
118. Birth trauma (22:35)
119. Kernicterus (22:35)
120. Hydrocephalus (22:35)
121. Birth anoxia (22:35)

A. Hemiplegia
B. Athetosis
C. Spastic paraparesis
D. Ataxia

Directions: For each of the following multiple choice questions, select the ONE most appropriate answer.

122. According to Eric Erikson, which period of one's life is crucial for the development of self?
A. infancy
B. toddler
C. childhood
D. adolescence (22:64)

123. Which one of the following is *not* true about disabled teen-agers?
A. they suffer substantial loss of self-esteem
B. loss of self-esteem is common if there are no other competency claims
C. they tend to limit their contacts to within their "protected" world
D. they use over-conformity and very orthodox attitudes to gain acceptance (22:62,65)

124. Which one of the following is *not* true about parents of a handicapped child?
A. they tend to limit socializing with other parents of disabled
B. parental participation in cerebral palsy organizations is greatest when diagnosis is first made
C. they are caught between embracing or ignoring their child's disability
D. they are generally willing to put their handicapped child in mixed situations to encourage them to develop like a nonhandicapped (22:66,67)

I. Convulsive Disorders

Directions: Match the following numbered items with the most appropriate lettered items.

125. Typified by the loss of consciousness, alternating tonic and clonic phases and post-seizure stupor (13:587)
126. Typified by period of unconsciousness accompanied by seemingly purposeful motor activity (13:587)

127. Typified by sudden involuntary muscle contractions of trunk and arms (13:587)
128. Usually involves muscles of hand, tongue, face and foot (13:587)
129. Also called tonoclonic seizure (13:587)
130. Poses the most difficult treatment problem (10:515)
131. Synonymous with jacksonian epilepsy (13:358)

A. Psychomotor seizure
B. A focal seizure
C. Grand mal seizure
D. Myoclonic seizure

Directions: For each of the following multiple choice questions, select the ONE most appropriate answer.

132. The epileptic episode typified by partial or complete loss of consciousness which is seen mainly in children is called
    A. jacksonian-march seizure
    B. grand mal seizure
    C. petit mal seizure
    D. myoclonic seizure (10:516)

133. What is the other name for autonomic epilepsy or seizure equivalents?
    A. status epilepticus
    B. psychomotor seizure
    C. abdominal epilepsy
    D. grand mal seizure (10:518)

134. A drug of choice for grand mal seizure is
    A. dilantin
    B. Valium
    C. phenobarbital
    D. Mysoline (13:588)

135. Which one of the following is true about epilepsy?
    A. EEG ("brain-wave") test can tell what the child's mentality is like
    B. children generally outgrow epilepsy
    C. medicines generally control many seizures, but there is no cure
    D. insanity and retardation cause epilepsy (13:588)

136. Which of the following types of diets is frequently ordered for epileptic patients?
    A. bland
    B. ketogenic
    C. low-salt
    D. low cholesterol (13:588)

137. What is the drug of choice in generalized and partial convulsive seizures?
    A. Mysoline
    B. phenobarbital
    C. dilantin
    D. Valium (10:521)

138. Which one of the following is *not* true about surgical treatment for epilepsy?
    A. surgery may bring about a cure if the epilepsy arises from one local area of the brain
    B. surgery is rarely used in small children except when a tremor is present
    C. surgery frequently cures even if the seizures affect both sides of the body
    D. surgical intervention is limited to patients who could not be satisfactorily controlled by any known anticonvulsant (10:522,523)

139. Ketogenic diet is clinically composed of
    A. two parts fat and two parts carbohydrate
    B. one part carbohydrate and two parts fat
    C. three parts fat and one part carbohydrate
    D. one part fat and three parts carbohydrate (13:588)

140. What should be the most important nursing role in the care of epileptic children?
    A. teaching the child to care for himself
    B. teaching the mother to care for her epileptic child
    C. teaching the child to recognize and report sore throats, fever and other signs of infections
    D. teaching the child to take anti-seizure medication on time (13:588)

141. Which of the following health teachings should be emphasized for children taking dilantin?
    A. avoid swimming alone
    B. daily brushing and massaging of the gums

C. limit physical activity
D. regular care of skin and eyes (13:588)

142. Which of the following actions is contraindicated in the care of a patient during an epileptic attack?
  A. if the patient is standing at the beginning of an attack, ease him down to the floor to prevent falling
  B. if he is on the floor, kneel and cradle his head in your lap or on a pillow
  C. hold him down to keep him from thrashing around
  D. if his teeth are not clenched, put a corner of a towel or a sleeve in between them (13:588)

143. Symptomatic epilepsy is defined as
  A. seizures with no known cause
  B. chronic, recurrent seizures which have sudden onset and a spontaneous resolution
  C. seizures resulting from cerebral lesions
  D. alternating clonic and tonic seizures (10:513)

144. Which of the following is *not* true about the incidence of epilepsy?
  A. 75% of all epileptic patients have an initial attack before 20 years of age
  B. 50% of all epileptics have an initial attack after 10 years of age
  C. an initial attack of petit mal epilepsy rarely occurs before age 2 or after age 12
  D. an initial seizure occurring after the age of 25 is indicative of status epilepticus (10:573)

145. If a school child should have a convulsive seizure while you are conversing, you should
  A. put something between his teeth
  B. move away furniture and hard objects
  C. ease him to floor and loosen collar
  D. turn his head to one side (5:121)

146. In order to answer questions that parents have about epilepsy, the nurse should know that
  1. meningitis and encephalitis may predispose a child to seizure
  2. cerebral anoxia may result in convulsive seizures
  3. convulsions in school-age children are commonly the result of a high fever
  4. convulsions are frequently caused by brain tumors in children
  A. 1 and 4
  B. 1 and 3
  C. 2 and 3
  D. 2 and 4 (13:586)

147. Which of the following symptoms is associated with the clonic phase of convulsion?
  A. fixed eyes
  B. twitching of extremities
  C. stiffening of body
  D. A and C (13:587)

The following are some principles that are found to be very valuable in the overall management of the epileptic patient. The choices are exemplifications of the principle.

Directions: Match the following numbered items with the most appropriate lettered items.

148. Patient and parental cooperation is very important (19:13)
149. Routine follow-up visits are a most important aspect of treatment (19:13)
150. Proper dosage should control seizures without interfering with well-being (19:22)
151. Treatment should be started with one drug (19:23)
152. Treatment should be instituted as soon as a diagnosis has been established (19:14)
153. Laboratory examinations should be carried out during the course of therapy (19:14)
154. Medication should be discontinued very gradually (19:41)

A. Sudden withdrawal of anticonvulsant drug is a frequent cause of recurrence of seizures
B. Intoxication may result from concurrent use of some drugs
C. It is considerably difficult to determine the cause of some type of unknown

reaction when two or more drugs are initially prescribed
D. Symptoms and signs occurring during drug therapy should be reported promptly
E. Emphasize importance of taking medication regularly and precisely as prescribed
F. Early treatment aids control
G. Check all patients thoroughly for signs and symptoms of intracranial neoplasm
H. Drug dosage varies with individuals

Directions: For each of the following multiple choice questions, select the ONE most appropriate answer.

155. An adverse effect of dilantin, which can cause a very serious cosmetic problem for female adolescents, is
    A. alopecia
    B. hypertrichosis
    C. obesity
    D. ecchymosis   (19:16)

156. A side effect of dilantin is
    A. diplopia
    B. vertigo
    C. hematuria
    D. marked drowsiness   (19:13)

157. A side effect of Mysoline is
    A. diplopia
    B. vertigo
    C. hematuria
    D. marked drowsiness   (19:13)

158. Another name for Mysoline is
    A. Reserpin
    B. Ritalin
    C. primidone
    D. diphenylhydantoin sodium   (19:13)

159. The use of dilantin for the control of epileptic seizures is specifically contraindicated in the following, *except*
    A. infants
    B. young adults
    C. adolescent females
    D. children receiving orthodontic treatment   (19:15)

160. A common sign and symptom of phenylhydantoin intoxication in infants, which is exceedingly difficult to recognize, is
    A. ataxia
    B. hypertrichosis
    C. marked drowsiness
    D. gingival hyperplasia   (19:15)

Directions: This part of the test consists of a situation followed by a series of statements or questions. Study the situation and select the best answer to each statement or question that follows.

Situation: Jane Barber, a 15-month-old child, was brought to the emergency room by her mother after the child had "a spell of unconsciousness and twitching." She had been ill for two days and was listless and not eating. The family doctor had seen her that afternoon and ordered penicillin. The child awoke crying and fretful. Her mother picked her up. The child became stiff, her eyes fixed and she had twitching of her right and left arms. The seizure lasted for about 15 minutes, and Jane fell asleep. In the emergency room, Jane was drowsy. Her temperature was 102° F. Mrs. Barber said that her child never acted like this before.

161. There are numerous causes for convulsive seizures in children this age. From the history recorded, the most likely cause of the seizure was
    A. a hard bump on the head from a previous fall
    B. low blood sugar due to her illness
    C. an infection with an elevated temperature
    D. increased intracranial pressure from an infection   (10:514)

162. From the physical examination, the doctor locates a bulging ear drum and an inflamed pharynx. He suspects that the associated otitis media originated from the pharyngitis. What anatomical finding(s) in this age child support(s) this suspicion? The eustachian tube
    A. has a mucous membrane lining continuous to that in the pharynx and middle ear
    B. is shorter, wider and straighter in chil-

Developmental Problems

dren this age than in older children and adults
C. has its opening adjacent to the adenoids, which are usually infected in pharyngitis
D. all of the above (13:329)

163. Jane is to be admitted. You are to prepare a crib for her. Knowing about convulsive seizures you should
A. pad the sides of the crib to prevent injury
B. provide a padded tongue blade to prevent tongue biting
C. provide a soft pillow to keep head from arching
D. A and B (13:589)

164. If you are observing a convulsive seizure, which of the following observations would be *least* important to record as related to neurologic etiology?
A. parts of body involved and where seizure began
B. eye movements and pupillary changes
C. amount and type of vomitus
D. length of seizure and posture of body (13:587)

165. If you were to advise the mother about what to do if she observes the start of a seizure, you would *stress*
A. inserting a soft object between Jane's teeth
B. holding Jane tightly to prevent injury
C. holding Jane in a sitting position to improve breathing
D. A and B (13:589)

166. Which of the following is not a common cause of fever in children?
A. immature nervous system
B. infection
C. dehydration
D. allergy (13:402)

167. Early and effective reduction of fever in children is quite important because prolonged fever precipitates
A. brain cell necrosis
B. convulsions
C. Down's syndrome
D. A and B (10:206,207)

168. Increased loss of body heat through evaporation is associated with the following physiological changes, *except*
A. dilation of peripheral blood vessels
B. constriction of peripheral blood vessels
C. increased respirations
D. increased secretion of sweat glands (13:336)

169. Which of the following nursing measures is *inappropriate* for the management of a highly febrile child?
A. sponge the child with equal parts alcohol and water
B. apply mild friction to the child's skin surface
C. wrap the child in wet clothes
D. increase the child's fluid intake (13:403)

J. Hyperkinetic Behavior Syndrome

Directions: For each of the following **multiple choice** questions, select the **ONE** most appropriate answer.

170. Which of the following statements is true about hyperkinetic behavior syndrome?
A. it is synonymous with overactivity
B. it is a specific combination of behaviors resulting from anything which can produce dysfunction of diencephalon and diencephalocortical interrelations
C. it is found in children of low levels of intelligence
D. it is a common manifestation of mental retardation (18:15)

171. Another name for hyperkinetic behavior syndrome is
A. hyperactivity
B. communication dysfunction
C. minimal brain dysfunction
D. hyperkinetic impulse disorder (18:15,16)

172. Which of the following symptoms and signs is *not a* characteristic of the child with the hyperkinetic impulse disorder?
    A. impulsiveness and inability to delay gratification
    B. preservation
    C. overactivity
    D. short attention span and poor powers of attention (18:16)

173. Which one of the signs below is most clinically important in establishing the impression of hyperkinetic impulse disorder?
    A. short attention span and poor power of attention — seen by teacher
    B. hyperactivity
    C. preservation
    D. variability, irritability and explosiveness (18:16)

174. Which of the following activity variables is *least helpful* in differentiating a child with hyperkinetic impulse disorder and normal children?
    A. quality
    B. intensity
    C. persistence
    D. quantity (18:16)

175. Babies reflecting hyperkinetic impulse disorders (HID) will show the following manifestations, *except*
    A. excessive jumpiness
    B. overreaction to light, noise and other stimuli
    C. extreme querulousness
    D. none of the above (18:16)

176. Which of the following statements is true about hyperactive babies? Such babies
    A. may lag in speech and language development
    B. may walk and talk early, reflecting advanced motor and language development
    C. always have sleeping problems
    D. lag behind in personal-social behavior (18:19)

177. Hyperkinetic children have low self-esteem. In planning for activities designed primarily for self-image building, which one of the following would be *least* helpful?
    A. model building
    B. music lessons
    C. crafts
    D. puzzles (18:27)

178. A part of the brain which plays an important role in programming behavior is the
    A. frontal lobe
    B. temporal lobe
    C. occipital lobe
    D. parietal lobe (18:32)

179. In dealing with hyperkinetic children, the nurse should primarily be
    A. flexible and considerate
    B. firm but loving and fair
    C. patient and tolerant of their impulsiveness
    D. unstructured in planning activities (18:59)

180. In parental counseling, the nurse should impress upon the parents the following points, *except* the fact that
    A. since many hyperkinetic children have poor time concepts and are forgetful, punishment is meaningless
    B. whenever possible, situations which are unfamiliar, noisy, stimulating, and/or sedentary for long periods should be avoided
    C. since hyperactive children have difficulty judging and appraising situations, useful habits must be stressed so that reflex reactions to a situation will be socially acceptable ones
    D. tasks should be initially presented globally then broken down into parts (18:58–61)

181. When a hyperkinetic child is under behavior modification therapy, the nurse understands this as
    A. establishing complete unilaterality of motor dominance for eye, hand, and foot
    B. advocating the administration of large doses of vitamins

C. advocating immediate reinforcement of quiet behavior
D. stressing the importance of low levels of glucose, histimine, and trace minerals (18:63)

182. In isolating a screaming, kicking hyperactive child, it is essentially important to remember that keeping a child isolated for too long would be a mistake because
   A. prolonged inactivity will eventually make him very uncooperative
   B. undue isolation will only make him hate the disciplining adult
   C. excess of enforced inactivity may then "charge him up" again
   D. isolation will never do him any good (18:61)

183. Hyperactive children almost universally have
   A. low self-esteem
   B. low intelligence
   C. poor motor coordination
   D. perceptual disturbances (18:61)

184. Which of the following statements is *not* true about the use of drug therapy for hyperkinetic children?
   A. the use of drugs and their actions upon hyperactive children still remains vague
   B. the stimulant drugs tend to quiet and subdue behavior in hyperactive children
   C. there is conclusive evidence at present that learning abilities and motor skills are significantly altered by stimulant drugs
   D. cerebral stimulants are the best drugs for beginning therapy (18:61)

185. The generic name for Thorazine is
   A. chlorpromazine
   B. dextroamphetamine
   C. methylphenidate
   D. thioridazine (18:71)

186. The trade name for methylphenidate is
   A. Dexedrine
   B. Millaril
   C. Miltown
   D. Ritalin (18:71)

Situation: A mother asks you how she could teach Billy to "get her a glass of water." "I simply could not get this simple instruction through to him." Match the numbered phrase with its appropriate place in the sequence of instructions.

187. Take a glass from the cupboard (18:86)
188. Turn on the faucet (18:86)
189. Put the glass under the faucet (18:86)
190. Go to the kitchen (18:86)
191. Bring the filled glass to me (18:86)
192. When the glass is filled, turn off the faucet (18:86)

   A. First step
   B. Second step
   C. Third step
   D. Fourth step
   E. Fifth step
   F. Sixth step

K. Mental Retardation

Directions: For each of the following multiple choice questions, select the ONE most appropriate answer.

193. The numbered items are various causes of mental retardation. With which of these causes is there a specific therapeutic regimen which, if instituted promptly and properly, may prevent severe retardation?
   1. congenital hypothyroidism
   2. trisomy—21
   3. phenylketonuria
   4. galactosemia
   5. microcephaly
      A. 1, 3 and 4
      B. 1, 3 and 5
      C. 2, 4 and 5
      D. all of the above (13:589)

194. Which of the following observations might lead you to suspect that a 6-month-old child is mentally retarded?
   A. flattened occipitus
   B. does not pursue toy when dropped
   C. unable to sit unsupported even for brief periods
   D. all of the above (13:589)

195. Why is it important to check the head circumference frequently during the first two years of life?
    A. the adult brain size is reached within this time period
    B. deviations greater than 2 standard deviations result in brain damage
    C. rapid brain growth normally occurs during this time
    D. B and C   (28:6)

196. What principle should you follow in interacting with a child who is mentally retarded?
    A. developmental age should determine how the child is treated
    B. try to treat the child as you would a normal child of that age
    C. provide an environment that is appropriate for the child to meet developmental milestones on schedule
    D. if the child appears happy and can be described as a "good" child, you can be assured her needs are being met
                                            (13:591)

197. You are the nurse helping a family teach a mentally retarded child to perform certain developmental tasks. Which of the following would you suggest?
    1. following a definite routine
    2. repeating the task over and over
    3. selecting a task above his level of ability to challenge him
    4. maintaining a relaxed but varied approach
    A. 1 and 2
    B. 1 and 3
    C. 2 and 4
    D. 3 and 4   (13:591)

Directions: This part of the test consists of a situation followed by a series of statements or questions. Study the situation and select the best answer to each statement or question that follows.

Situation: George Martin, age 6, was referred to the school psychologist for assessment by the school nurse. His teachers stated that he could not count the number of fingers on one hand and could not add beyond the sum of one and one. He had been able to keep up with the learning experiences marginally during kindergarten, but was not doing passing work in first grade. His school records indicate that he had encephalitis at 9 months of age. According to the American Association on Mental Deficiency, George can be referred to as mentally retarded.

198. Which of the following is *not* one of the criteria used in the definition?
    A. demonstration of subaverage intellectual functioning
    B. originating during childhood development between conception to age 16
    C. symptom etiology of encephalitis
    D. impairment of adaptive behavior
                                            (7:464)

199. George was classified as trainable with an I.Q. of 38. Which of the following behaviors could be projected for him?
    A. will probably respond to traditional education in writing
    B. can probably be capable of competitive employment
    C. will probably require supervision in personal matters
    D. may function in the community but will require custodial care at night   (7:465)

200. Which of the following is *not* a type of classification for mental retardation?
    A. learning handicap
    B. symptom etiology
    C. symptom severity
    D. clinical types   (7:468)

201. Mary Evans, a 10-year-old, trainable, mentally retarded child, was enrolled in the social rehabilitation workshop at the state school. She should be able to learn all of the following behaviors *except*
    A. setting the table
    B. serving lunch
    C. receiving payment for services rendered
    D. making correct change for customers
                                            (7:467)

202. Which of the following is *not* a possible etiology for mental retardation?
    A. congenital maternal intoxication

B. cultural familial retardation
C. birth anoxia
D. cystic fibrosis (7:464)

203. Which of the following is a true statement about the educable mentally retarded child?
A. he is not limited in the kinds of vocational choices that he can make
B. he will have discernible physical traits distinguishing him
C. motor skills proceed with a noticeable lag in rate
D. sequence of development is opposite of other children (7:465)

204. Which of the following would not be a factor related to the higher incidence of mental retardation in families living in poverty?
A. lack of prenatal care
B. poor nutrition
C. defective genetic components in such families
D. cultural deprivation (15:241)

205. Mrs. Thomas, mother of Suzy, a 5-year-old retarded girl, cried after the nurse indicated that Suzy was still functioning at the level previously tested 11 months ago. Mrs. Thomas said, "But, Miss Drew, I've worked and worked with Suzy, she just isn't trying!" Suzy turned her head away and threw a block at the wall. Which of the following would be the nurse's best response?
A. "I know you must feel disappointed, but Suzy will progress at her own rate of development."
B. "I understand how difficult it is to work with a child like Suzy."
C. "Have you followed the program we at the clinic established for you and Suzy?"
D. "I think you are pushing Suzy too hard, that is why she is so angry now."
(15:244)

206. Harvey Davis, a moderately retarded 13-year-old boy, is 5′ 10″ and 160 pounds. He is extremely active and has accidentally knocked over other children at his school. He is occasionally belligerent with his peers. Ingestion of which of the following could be part of his treatment?
A. vitamin C
B. Ritalin
C. phenobarbital
D. chlorpromazine (15:246)

207. Which of the following is a rationale for the use of operant conditioning in the treatment of mentally retarded children?
A. it enables the individual to modify behavior patterns through motivation
B. it is flexible, therefore failure can be ignored, decreasing frustration on the part of the retarded individual
C. the individual receives support from the peer group who help him set limits to his behavior
D. it has been found that the use of punishment as a negative reinforcer is especially successful with retarded children (15:247)

208. Which of the following best describes the aim of educational programs provided for mentally retarded children?
A. programs are designed to provide vocational guidance for retarded children
B. programs are designed to equip mentally retarded children to live as independently as possible
C. programs will teach all children toilet training and self-care skills
D. programs will enable retarded children to function in the community (15:250)

209. Which of the following best describes the nursing role in an institution for mentally retarded children?
A. provision of custodial care
B. maintenance of discipline
C. provision of mothering figure
D. health teaching (15:250)

210. At the public health well-child conference, Mrs. Johnson expressed concern about Joey who is four. She said, "He just isn't doing the things his older sister did at his

age. Do you think there is something wrong?" The nurse's best response would be to say
A. "Children sometimes develop at individual rates; however, I'll administer a Denver Developmental Test to see how he functions in comparison to most children his own age."
B. "Children develop at their own rates; let me administer an I.Q. test to see if it is normal for his age."
C. "That can really be a worry. I can administer the Denver Developmental Test to see if his I.Q. is within normal limits."
D. "I can understand that this might concern you. I'll make an appointment with our clinical psychologist who is our staff person qualified to do Denver Developmental testing." (7:476)

211. Nurse Merrick wishes to teach Johnny, a trainable 11-year-old mentally retarded child, about his need for bathing. Which of the following concepts should the nurse use in developing her teaching plan?
A. Johnny will only be able to learn the behavior if he is given adequate abstract explanation
B. the learning experience should encompass one protracted learning session rather than frequent brief intervals
C. the practice sessions should only occur in the presence of the nurse-teacher
D. retarded children respond to concrete ideas and objects best (7:476)

212. Which of the following is a specific characteristic found in group therapy with mentally retarded individuals that is not seen in normal group therapy sessions?
A. greater structure
B. peers exercise greater influence than the group leader
C. focus is on ideas rather than actions
D. fewer limits are required (15:247)

Chapter IV: Answers and Explanations

1. **C.**—Mummy restraints are used with infants and young children during treatment and examinations involving the head and neck.
2. **B.**—The nurse is responsible for positioning the infant so that blood can be drawn with the least difficulty for the physician and the least discomfort for the child.
3. **D.**—The regulation of drops should be done when infant is resting quietly. The flow should be carefully regulated to avoid circulatory overload.
4. **D.**—The nurse must be alert to observing increased respiration as this condition can readily lead to fatal cardiac embarrassment.
5. **A.**—Speeding up I.V. rate beyond the ordered rate of flow is extremely dangerous; it can readily cause a circulatory overload. An infant can tolerate up to 150 cc per kilogram of body weight per day in a continuous infusion.
6. **B.**—One cubic centimeter is equal to 60 microdrops.
7. **A.**—The frequency of voiding should be recorded. Although the amount cannot be measured, it should be estimated.
8. **B.**—The pH drops below 7.35 in cases of acidosis.
9. **D.**—Dryness of the mouth and loss of weight are other signs of dehydration.
10. **D.**—The nurse should only be concerned with relevant data.
11. **A.**—Undue stimulation of intestines could be initiated through irritation of the rectum by a rectal thermometer.
12. **C.**—Nurses should teach the mother proper isolation technique including the correct handwashing technique. The mother should be supported in her desire to care for her infant.
13. **B.**—The additional blankets should also be tucked in about his body.
14. **D.**—This is a very important precaution lest the patient gets burned.
15. **A.**—Forcing fluids is to be discouraged because such action too frequently leads to vomiting of all fluid taken.
16. **B.**—If the concentration of hydrogen ions is increased, the solution becomes more acid; if the concentration is decreased, it becomes more alkaline.
17. **A.**—If the pH of body fluid rises above 7.7 the patient's life is in danger.
18. **A.**—Solutes refer to the dissolved substance and solvent refers to the liquid dissolving the substance.
19. **C.**—The main portion of potassium which is exchangeable is intracellular.
20. **B.**—Sodium and chloride are the most important cation and anion of extracellular fluid. Sodium primarily functions in regulatory osmotic pressure, muscle and nerve irritability. Sodium has its major function in osmotic pressure.
21. **B.**—Metabolic acidosis is associated with a loss of bicarbonate from the extracellular fluid.
22. **C.**—The infant's extracellular fluid is approximately ⅓ of his body weight.
23. **A.**—Water intoxication occurs when *extracellular* fluid is replaced too rapidly.
24. **A.**—Strict isolation is necessary to protect the other children and personnel in the area as well as the members of the family at home.
25. **B.**—Since the child's intake would be strictly regimented, keeping the volume of ingested fluids down to, and within the volumes prescribed, can never be overemphasized.

26. **D.**—Without treatment the infant acquires the typical appearance of the starved child. He looks like a little man.
27. **B.**—With the increase in the plasma carbon dioxide content and in pH, there is a corresponding decrease in serum chloride.
28. **C.**—If medication is to be administered, it would indicate an antispasmodic drug instead of anticholinergic.
29. **A.**—This position should ordinarily disappear by the fourth month.
30. **D.**—Billy, at this point in time, would need sufficient bodily contact for sensory input, which would greatly influence his later perception of the world around him.
31. **B.**—Since the greater curvature of the stomach is towards the left side of the abdomen, placing the infant on the right side in elevated position would thus relieve the stomach of undue pressure.
32. **C.**—There is greater danger of aspirating vomitus when one is lying flat on his back.
33. **C.**—Treatments should never be given *just before, during* or *after* feeding time, since the situation is likely to produce tension which can stimulate vomiting.
34. **A.**—The causes of rumination are not known. It may be due to environmental tension or dislike of food or the person feeding the child.
35. **D.**—Alkalosis due to severe vomiting is due to a loss of chlorides and potassium.
36. **C.**—Clearing the airway should be done first to make sure that it is free of any mechanical obstruction.
37. **B.**—Keeping the mouth clean and free from irritation is extremely important. All strain on the sutures must be prevented.
38. **B.**—A straw, nipple or syringe should not be used for this would stimulate Michael to suck thereby straining the sutures.
39. **A.**—The foot of his bed may be elevated to further prevent aspiration of drainage material.
40. **A.**—For some reason, cleft palate is more common in girls than in boys; and cleft lip occurs more frequently among boys than among girls.
41. **A.**—It is thus important to instruct mothers to report any indication of otitis media and to learn the correct method of brushing the child's teeth; then she could teach the child the correct technique.
42. **D.**—A sympathetic, tactful nurse can do a great deal to relieve their distress.
43. **A.**—The surgeon's discussion of therapy with the parents is helpful in facilitating their adjustment to the newborn's malformation.
44. **C.**—Periodic arm exercises improve the blood circulation to the restrained limbs and can make Jimmy feel more comfortable.
45. **D.**—Cleft lip does not involve damage to the neck or to any of the structures controlling neck mobility.
46. **A.**—The aforenoted measures point out the special needs of a child following repair of the cleft palate.
47. **C.**—Bowel and bladder functioning also require careful evaluation.
48. **D.**—It is also important to help restore function orthopedically and urologically.
49. **B.**—The infant thus becomes increasingly helpless and less able to raise his head.
50. **B.**—Fixation in the correct position is important. The child should not be placed on his back, since such position would cause pressure on the sac.
51. **A.**—The goal of surgical treatment is closure of the surface defect while preserving all functioning nervous tissue.
52. **D.**—Abdominal distention caused by paralytic ileus or distention of the bladder follows most spinal cord surgery and should be reported immediately.
53. **B.**—The importance of coordination of all health services must be stressed and the nurse often acts as the coordinator.
54. **D.**—Frequent change of position is primarily for purposes of preventing hypostatic pneumonia and pressure sores.
55. **C.**—There is no disturbance in protein metabolism in cystic fibrosis; the deficiency is in fat absorption.
56. **B.**—Fats are very poorly absorbed in cystic fibrosis, therefore some other source of vitamins must be provided.
57. **D.**—Aerosol helps remove heavy secretions from the bronchi and relieves dyspnea, therefore it is best to give it just

Developmental Problems

before postural drainage and at least half an hour before meals.

58. **C.**—On the contrary, three children in the family will be normal, one a homozygous normal and two will be heterozygous normal.

59. **A.**—Absence of trypsin in the stool is indicative of cystic fibrosis.

60. **A.**—Good nutrition is essential. The patient should receive a balanced diet including a large amount of protein and sufficient amount of fat.

61. **D.**—Conferences with parents should provide for continuation of the care the child receives in the hospital.

62. **D.**—It is quite important to familiarize the patient with the equipment used in potentially traumatic procedures to lessen her anxiety.

63. **B.**—Susan's developmental level is likely to be below that of an average 3-year-old.

64. **D.**—Cutting out paper dolls or jumping rope would be activities too advanced for Susan. Playing with windmills would predispose her to inhale sand or dust.

65. **C.**—Cough medicine would be given only upon physician's orders; codeine and terpin hydrate are contraindicated in infancy.

66. **C.**—For this reason, the diabetic child and his parents must be helped in developing positive attitudes toward the child's condition.

67. **D.**—Exercise produces a lowering of the blood sugar level and may cause shock in children taking insulin.

68. **C.**—The child should be stabilized on his diet and the amount of insulin he needs.

69. **D.**—The diabetic adolescent should be encouraged to participate on an equal basis with his peer group, not looking upon his diabetes as a handicap.

70. **B.**—The nurse should watch for changes in skin color, respiration and degree of consciousness.

71. **C.**—The child should carry a lump of sugar with him and once he recognizes symptoms of shock, take the sugar.

72. **B.**—Diabetic acidosis is associated with low CO_2 combining power.

73. **A.**—Bring child to normal adulthood through understanding of his problem.

74. **B.**—The child and his parents should recognize the need for immediate assistance if symptoms of shock or acidosis occur.

75. **C.**—The dose of insulin is estimated on the basis of quantitative tests of the urine for sugar.

76. **A.**—Polyuria may be the cause of bed-wetting in children who have achieved night control of urination.

77. **B.**—Parents should recognize that diabetic children basically have the same needs as any other children of their own age group. The diabetic adolescent needs support and understanding, particularly in dietary control, since his need to be like his peers is substantially great at this time. He may eat what they eat even though he knows he should not do so.

78. **A.**—Taking an interest in religion is an expression of the adolescent's developing sense of identity.

79. **B.**—Adolescence may be a difficult period for the diabetic youth and for his parents.

80. **D.**—If a free diet is ordered, the child will have little problem in controlling his food intake. He must be conditioned to self-control if a measured diet is ordered.

81. **D.**—Adolescence is the period in which a sense of identity and a sense of intimacy develop.

82. **D.**—Autistic children withdraw from contact with people in their environment. This is commonly seen between the third and fifth years, but may be seen as early as the second year.

83. **B.**—One should try to understand the child and his behavior, but the fantasy world which the child sees should never be reinforced.

84. **D.**—The schizophrenic individual usually has not learned to trust others and has not developed a self-image that make it possible for him to feel secure in interpersonal relations.

85. **C.**—Many authorities believe that it is related to factors that are inherent in highly complex cultures.

86. **D.**—Kanner's efforts led to formulation of theories explaining autistic behavior and consequently led to detailed studies of actual behavior of autistic children.

87. **C.**—Not all autistic children scream a great deal; some are content to lie quietly all day.
88. **B.**—Withdrawal from human contact is most frequently observed in children between 3 and 5 years of age although it may be seen as early as the second year.
89. **B.**—Autistic children explore their world through their senses of touch, taste and smell, and they do this long after the toddler stage has passed.
90. **C.**—Autistic children often make verbal mistakes because they cannot easily remember words.
91. **D.**—Autistic children hardly ever muddle the order of words inside sentences primarily because they have difficulty learning in complete sentences.
92. **C.**—Most young autistic children behave as though other people do not exist.
93. **A.**—Many autistic children insist on repetition of the same routines. Resistance to change can apply to food and some can go through a stage in which they eat only two kinds of food.
94. **D.**—Autistic children do not understand why it should ever be necessary to avoid the truth; they are very naive about social conventions and other people's feelings.
95. **B.**—Autistic children commonly have problems when they try to copy movements made by other people.
96. **B.**—Autistic children tend to become more affectionate and sociable but still resistant to change.
97. **C.**—The Montessori type exploits the use of touch and movement for learning and encourages social mixing within a structured environment.
98. **A.**—No studies to date have shown that autistic children have been raised in institutions void of emotionally supportive care.
99. **C.**—Ignoring the child without eventful reward is worthless when dealing with autistic children.
100. **B.**—Autistic children are especially prone to be upset by failure; hence, making sure that the child can succeed with each small stage is a good way of avoiding this problem.
101. **D.**—Such a task is excellent since there is nothing to break if the child drops something. Also, it involves remembering and naming each person in the family who has a place at the table. Each has the same implements and this gives the child an opportunity to learn to use and understand the words "knife," "fork," and "spoon."
102. **C.**—Preparing the child in advance through words and phrases may give familiarity to the situation, thus preventing him from being completely bewildered by the new surroundings.
103. **D.**—Asking questions about conception and birth presupposes a reasonable level of cognitive development which is hardly attained by autistic adolescents.
104. **C.**—It is estimated that there are close to half a million children suffering from cerebral palsy in the United States.
105. **D.**—The nonprogressive nature of cerebral lesion implies that no active disease process is in existence at the time the diagnosis is made.
106. **A.**—The motor function disorder is secondary to a static brain lesion that has occurred prenatally, perinatally, or postnatally.
107. **C.**—Cerebral palsy may be caused by the interplay of multiple factors.
108. **C.**—Children with spastic cerebral palsy comprise 50–60% of all the clinical types.
109. **A.**—A generalized hypotonia is seen in affected extremities. Early motor milestones are generally delayed by 5 to 6 months.
110. **D.**—The Moro and tonic neck reflex are retained often throughout the child's life span.
111. **C.**—It must be recognized that these factors are theoretical speculations.
112. **B.**—A large number of these patients have a rather severe neuromuscular dysfunction.
113. **C.**—Only about ½ of cerebral palsy children have some type of seizure disorder.
114. **B.**—Deafness and hearing loss are particularly of the higher frequencies.
115. **D.**—Drugs for treatment of motor dysfunction seem to have limited applicability. There is no standard drug therapy followed in the medical management of cerebral palsy.
116. **A.**—The parents should be helped out in handling their feelings about having borne

Developmental Problems

117. **C.**—The spastic paraparesis type has been associated with prematurity.
118. **A.**—Birth trauma tends to cause the hemiplegic type.
119. **B.**—Kernicterus has been associated with the athetosis type.
120. **D.**—The ataxia type is commonly seen in hydrocephalic children.
121. **B.**—The athetosis type has also been associated with birth anoxia.
122. **D.**—The adolescent period is the crucial stage for the development of one's sense of identity.
123. **C.**—Young people with cerebral palsy have been observed to seek out mixed social groups, as they consider this necessary for proving that they could handle difficult encounters as well as protected ones.
124. **D.**—Parents of cerebral palsy children have been observed to avoid putting their child in mixed situations, not only to protect the child, but also to avoid having to explain the child's condition to the outside world.
125. **C.**—Grand mal seizures in children are not likely to be preceded by an aura common in adults.
126. **A.**—As such, psychomotor seizures cannot be recognized easily.
127. **D.**—This type of seizure is usually accompanied by mental retardation.
128. **B.**—A focal seizure begins in one area of the body and spreads to other areas on the same side in a fixed pattern.
129. **C.**—The seizure is a generalized convulsion; a tonic phase and a clonic phase are seen.
130. **D.**—Since frequent seizures may result in regression, differentiation from primary cerebral degenerative diseases is difficult.
131. **B.**—Jacksonian epilepsy may be either motor or sensory.
132. **C.**—Petit mal seizure is also called absence attack or pyknolepsy.
133. **C.**—This type is thought to be a form of focal epilepsy characterized by paroxysmal abdominal pain.
134. **A.**—Dilantin is an effective anticonvulsant but does not produce excessive drowsiness as barbiturates may.
135. **C.**—Many parents know that there is no cure for epilepsy but they want to believe that there is one.
136. **B.**—A ketogenic diet and a reduction of fluid intake tend to prevent seizures.
137. **B.**—Phenobarbital is perhaps the single drug which may be used for all types of seizures.
138. **C.**—Drug and diet therapies are most commonly imposed.
139. **B.**—The diet should be varied and palatable since a ketogenic diet, containing large amounts of fat, is not too appetizing.
140. **D.**—The importance of taking drugs on time should be emphasized.
141. **B.**—Painless hypertrophy of the gums may follow administration of dilantin.
142. **C.**—Such action is likely to cause fractures of long bones.
143. **C.**—The attacks are classified as partial because the abnormal discharge begins over one cerebral hemisphere.
144. **D.**—Seizure types change, depending on the age at onset. In general, the younger the age at onset, the more serious the lesion.
145. **C.**—Prevent child from hitting his head against a hard surface while at the same time not restraining the jerking.
146. **A.**—The aforenoted factors may cause organic epilepsy whereby degenerative changes may take place in the brain.
147. **B.**—The clonic phase, which consists of alternate relaxation and contraction of muscles, lasts indefinitely. This is then followed by a deep sleep.
148. **E.**—Patient and parents should recognize that with understanding, cooperation and proper treatment, complete control of seizures can be attained.
149. **G.**—These check-ups are especially important for patients whose seizures started during late adolescence and early adulthood.
150. **H.**—Clinical response and blood drug level are the important criteria that doctors observe in regulating the dosage of anticonvulsant drugs.
151. **C.**—Other drugs are prescribed only after the maximal dose of the initial drug has

failed to produce satisfactory clinical response.
152. **F.**—The parents, or the patient, should be instructed to report promptly any sign or symptom not present before the drug was prescribed.
153. **D.**—Careful check-ups are necessary to be alerted readily to any adverse drug effects.
154. **A.**—The period necessary for complete withdrawal is governed by the severity of the patient's previous seizure state and by dosage.
155. **B.**—The abnormal growth of hair persists to some degree in all patients after discontinuation of the drug.
156. **A.**—Diplopia is double vision.
157. **C.**—It is important to familiarize the patient with the expected effects of drugs prescribed for him.
158. **D.**—Mysoline is the second drug of choice for grand mal epilepsy.
159. **B.**—Dilantin causes a lot of adverse reactions, such as gingival hyperplasia and hypertrichosis.
160. **A.**—Thus, infants on phenylhydantoin must be placed under close observation.
161. **C.**—Febrile convulsions are the most common type of seizure in this age span.
162. **D.**—Otitis media is usually secondary to a respiratory infection.
163. **D.**—The patient must be protected from self-injury.
164. **C.**—Vomiting rarely accompanies a convulsive seizure.
165. **A.**—This measure is to prevent the child from biting her tongue.
166. **D.**—Allergy is rarely accompanied by fever. Common causes of acute fever of unknown origin are viral upper respiratory infections.
167. **D.**—During convulsions, there is a corresponding slowing down of oxygen supply to the brain cells with subsequent anoxia if the convulsion is prolonged. Death of the brain cells will then occur and the damage is irreversible.
168. **B.**—Constriction of peripheral blood vessels conserves body heat.
169. **C.**—Wrapping the child in wet clothes restricts evaporation thus slowing down the cooling process.
170. **B.**—This condition occurs usually before birth or in the first five years of life.
171. **D.**—Hyperkinetic children are often confused with autistic children.
172. **C.**—Overactivity refers to a normal desire of children to explore, while hyperactivity may be a sign of deprivation, frustration, disenchantment, rebellion or attention getting.
173. **A.**—The said signs are the ones most readily seen by teachers.
174. **D.**—It has been demonstrated that the activity of a hyperkinetic child does not differ in amount from that of a normal child.
175. **D.**—All the aforenoted signs describe hyperkinetic behavior.
176. **B.**—Hyperkinetic babies often have advanced developmental schedules.
177. **D.**—Puzzles call for a lot of concentration and hyperkinetic children can hardly be expected to do this.
178. **A.**—Studies have shown that destruction of the frontal lobe renders the organism unable to create dominant associations to control his behavior.
179. **B.**—Change in routine is very distressing to hyperkinetic children so that daily activities should be kept as stable and simple as possible.
180. **D.**—Tasks are better taught when broken into minute components and the components taught one at a time.
181. **C.**—Socially acceptable behavior should be reinforced immediately.
182. **C.**—Putting the child in a state of prolonged inactivity could be most frustrating and would just make the situation worse.
183. **A.**—Low self-esteem comes from frustration and doubt about his own ability and results from continued failure in athletic or academic achievements or in the inability to behave in a manner that results in praise.
184. **C.**—There is no conclusive evidence to that effect.
185. **A.**—Thorazine or chlorpromazine is sometimes preferred by physicians for hyperactive children who also manifest a high degree of anxiety, hostility or aggression.
186. **D.**—Ritalin may produce an increase in activity rather than the desired decrease,

Developmental Problems

but the most frequent side effects are anorexia and insomnia.

187. **B.**
188. **D.**
189. **C.**   There is a need to sensitize parents much more about this kind of communication. Hyperkinetic children are incapable of handling conventional methods of learning.
190. **A.**
191. **F.**
192. **E.**

193. **A.**—Mental retardation caused by phenylketonuria may be checked by a low phenylalanine diet.
194. **D.**—A diagnosis of mental retardation should be made only after a thorough study of the family and the child.
195. **C.**—After the second year, brain growth is slow and the adult brain size is reached at adolescence.
196. **A.**—The child needs to be treated according to his mental age regardless of his chronological age.
197. **A.**—Repetition and consistency are basic principles underlying any educational endeavor with the mentally retarded.
198. **C.**—This is a method of classification for mental retardation but is not used in the diagnosis of mental retardation.
199. **C.**—A trainable retardate can function in the community, but requires close supervision.
200. **A.**—Children with learning handicaps do not have the defined characteristics of the mentally retarded.
201. **D.**—This requires abstract thinking which is beyond the trainable mentally retarded child's level of cognition.
202. **D.**—Cystic fibrosis is not one of the conditions specified under symptom etiology by the American Association of Mental Deficiency.
203. **C.**—This is usually one of the signs which may indicate that this child is retarded.
204. **C.**—Defective genetic components are not limited to certain social classes.
205. **A.**—The nurse is giving support and yet is cautioning the mother against comparison of Suzy with her normal siblings. The other answers might underline the mother's sense of failure. Answer C seems to exclude the mother from any planning of Suzy's program at home.
206. **D.**—Chlorpromazine has proved helpful in quieting overactive, boisterous, excited mentally retarded children.
207. **A.**—The use of positive reinforcers such as praise, food, and privileges motivates the child to learn new behaviors or phase out undesirable behaviors.
208. **B.**—The extent of independence attained will depend upon the severity, symptom etiology, and individual and family resources, among other things. The other answers are incorrect because they are not realistic goals for all mentally retarded children.
209. **C.**—Because these children are removed from their families, they must establish other relationships to meet the needs previously met by the mother. The other roles are a part of the mothering role or extensions of it.
210. **A.**—This statement best explains the Denver Developmental Test which is appropriate for a nurse to administer (an I.Q. test is not), and also points out the individual differences in children to this mother.
211. **D.**—This is the level of cognition at which most retarded children are able to perform.
212. **A.**—This greater structure is required to provide security for the children and should be externally provided, as these children cannot structure the situation themselves.

CHAPTER V

Situational Problems and Their Nursing Care

INTRODUCTION

There is much current emphasis in health-care delivery systems on prevention, early diagnosis and early treatment of health problems. In order to participate in fulfilling this mandate, it is essential that the nurse possess a frame of reference from which to view the physiological and behavioral phenomena of health and illness. Awareness of the etiological factors, the psycho-physiological and psycho-social changes associated with health and illness should enable the nurse to maximize her professional potential in the delivery of health care.

Situational problems account for most of the health deviations and other handicapping complications from infancy through death. They pose several challenges to the health professions and critical issues to the health care delivery system. Nursing is called upon to play an all important role in health restoration. It is thus essential that the nurse have substantial knowledge of the complex correlations of the many factors underlying illness. Specifically, she must have a basic understanding of the etiological factors, diagnostic studies, clinical manifestations of different diseases, modes of treatment, and the potential responses of patients upon which she can intelligently base her nursing intervention.

Like the preceding chapter, the content herein is presented in situation and multiple-choice question format. Substantial attention is given to the impact of illness and hospitalization upon the child and the family, and pathophysiological considerations as well as nursing care. Attempts have been made to minimize the possibility of overloading you with confusing technical facts.

A. Hospitalization for Children

Directions: For each of the following multiple choice questions, select the ONE most appropriate answer.

1. In which of the following countries was rooming-in first practiced in children's hospitals?
   A. England
   B. United States
   C. Australia
   D. Israel (16:7)

2. Vaccinations against contagious diseases have brought about the following changes in the care of hospitalized children, *except*
   A. setting up of school rooms and children's departments
   B. setting up of playrooms for group recreation and play therapy
   C. using parents in care of child while hospitalized
   D. improvement of medical precautions and isolation techniques (16:7)

3. A child can be best prepared for hospital procedures by the following approaches *except*
   A. explaining to him ahead of time what procedures will take place
   B. giving him miniature equipment for him to use as dolls
   C. allowing him to see and touch equipment similar to that which will be used in the procedure
   D. taking him to zoo or children's movie a day before admission into the hospital
   (16:9)

4. Factors limiting the effectiveness of children's hospitalization include the following, *except*
   A. physical design of the ward
   B. participation of parents in care of child during hospitalization
   C. disruption of school and work
   D. separation from family (16:7,9,11)

5. Which of the following measures is *least* effective in reducing the need for hospitalization of children?
   A. provide insurance programs that only offer reimbursement for health care obtained in in-patient setting
   B. provide equal educational opportunities
   C. improve living conditions
   D. fight against pollution control (16:12)

6. Protecting the health of all children involves the provision of
   A. diagnostic facilities
   B. therapeutic facilities
   C. rehabilitative facilities
   D. all of the above (16:12)

7. In planning for architectural design of infant's units, one must take into account the needs and developmental tasks in the first year of life. These include the following, *except*
   A. basic physical care
   B. sensory and social stimulation
   C. toilet training
   D. development of motor skills (16:15)

8. Activities that could give infants visual, tactile and auditory stimulation and which could all be facilitated through physical design include the following, *except*
   A. touching and playing with water and food
   B. playing with checkers and marbles
   C. crawling on diverse floor textures
   D. watching changes of light and shadow
   (16:15)

9. Hospital design for toddlers and preschoolers should allow for
   A. adequate visual supervision of patients at all times
   B. freedom from equipment and construction likely to cause accidents
   C. opportunities for environmental exploration
   D. all of the above (16:16)

10. Of the following, which is the most important consideration for preschoolers and toddlers in the hospital?
    A. play space
    B. bathroom
    C. dining room
    D. treatment room (16:16)

11. Play areas in hospitals can be constructed in several ways. Which of the following is a risky measure?
    A. separate play areas designed to accommodate children in cribs, wheelchairs, beds, etc.
    B. make sleeping areas extra large so that play can take place there and can include children confined to bed
    C. set up outdoor play areas like those designed for healthy prekindergarten children
    D. none of the above (16:16)

12. Which of the following hospital conditions would be *least* beneficial to school-age children?
    A. facilities for continuity in exercise of cognitive, motor and artistic skills
    B. facilities for musical experience and for indoor and outdoor play

C. opportunities to live and work with others
D. a "secret" room (16:16)

13. Which of the following measures is *least* effective when caring for hospitalized children 3 to 7 years old?
    A. assigning one nurse to the child as consistently as possible
    B. encouraging mother's participation in child's care
    C. avoiding suggestions of damage and repair of construction toys
    D. encouraging participation in medical care and self-hygiene (16:32)

14. It is especially important to repeatedly reassure a school-age child that no one is to blame for his condition or hospitalization because
    A. a child in this age group is likely to be preoccupied with guilt and blame; he tends to generalize and feels that all body parts are vulnerable
    B. this will encourage him to ask questions about his illness, thereby facilitating self-understanding
    C. this will evoke a warm response from the child, thus facilitating rapport
    D. this will facilitate active participation in self-care (16:33)

15. Which of the following measures is a most important consideration when preparing a 4-year-old child for eye surgery?
    A. familiarize the child with eye patches and restraints
    B. play at recognizing voices and events in room with eyes closed
    C. arrange in advance for the continuous presence of a family member
    D. reassure child that no other part of the body will be operated on (16:33)

16. Which of the following activities would be most helpful to a 9-year-old boy who is recuperating following leg amputation?
    A. playing Chinese checkers with 2 other ambulatory boys
    B. watching television in the playroom
    C. drawing or painting about hospital experience
    D. reading comics (16:40)

17. Parents of a hospitalized child may be encouraged to photograph hospital scenes related to their child. What purposes do the photographs serve?
    A. to help child gain ego mastery of hospitalization
    B. to help enable child to clarify the difference between fantasy and reality in a hospital setting
    C. A and B
    D. none of the above (16:40)

18. Inviting a child to visit the unit after discharge
    A. provides staff with an opportunity to evaluate child's adjustment following hospitalization
    B. helps child maintain contacts with staff
    C. helps child correct distorted memories and diminishes anxiety in event of future hospitalization
    D. all of the above (16:41)

19. Which of the following factors has the *least* influence upon the impact of hospitalization on children's behavior?
    A. timing and duration of stress
    B. interdisciplinary team approach
    C. strength child brings to situation
    D. quality and quantity of support given by parents and child care workers (16:41)

20. Hospitalized children between the ages of seven months and five years are developmentally vulnerable and psychologically at risk. Which of the following does *not* support this contention?
    A. they cannot be prepared through verbal or play approaches
    B. their defense repertoires and memories are inadequate to sustain
    C. they need a mother's presence to sustain development and avoid emotional trauma
    D. the child cannot master his anxieties by himself (16:45)

21. Play in the hospital enables the child to achieve the following *except*
    A. continue with as many aspects of normal growth as possible
    B. place his hospital experience in understandable and tolerable context
    C. communicate his concerns and fears, facilitating treatment
    D. mask his anxiety and other coping behaviors (16:45)

22. Which of the following principles is *least* effective when preparing a child for hospitalization?
    A. give factual, honest information to arm child with knowledge of what will happen to and around him
    B. fortify or establish a relation between child and available adult whom he can trust
    C. require child's mother to stay with child in hospital
    D. encourage child to participate actively, verbalize his questions, and express his emotions (16:45)

23. The chief trauma of hospitalization for the young child is frequently the
    A. exposure to strange people
    B. separation from his mother or mother surrogate
    C. exposure to strange environment
    D. change of routines of daily living (10:140)

24. The adverse impact of hospitalization on the adolescent is generally brought about by
    A. separation from family
    B. separation from peer group
    C. absence from school
    D. enforced passivity and dependency during illness (16:141)

25. Parents also need opportunities to discuss their own anxieties. Which of the following tasks may *not* counteract a mother's feelings of helplessness?
    A. complete questionnaire about child's preferences
    B. read materials to her child concerning admission procedures and typical hospital activities
    C. "rap" sessions with other parents
    D. read child's hospital chart (16:141)

26. Which of the following best describes the preparation of children for hospitalization?
    A. preparation is a process which continues through last day of admission into hospital
    B. preparation of child offers an opportunity to minimize emotional trauma of hospitalization
    C. information which reduces fears can be given by physicians, nurses and parents, from books, pamphlets and movies
    D. timing and content of preparation must be matched to needs of child (16:142)

27. Which of the following is *not* a basic difference between children's response to illness and the response of adults?
    A. children become seriously ill much more quickly than do adults
    B. children are relatively defenseless
    C. children are constantly changing and, as such, are predictable
    D. children get more readily dehydrated than do adults (13:41)

28. Which of the following play activities would be best suited to a 2-year-old boy on prolonged bed rest?
    1. watching a plant, such as a carrot or vine grow
    2. watching some goldfish in a tank
    3. watching supervised television programs
    4. finger painting
    A. 1 and 2
    B. 2 and 4
    C. all except 4
    D. all of the above (13:59)

29. Which of the following activities should be encouraged for a 3-year-old hospitalized child suffering from separation anxiety?
    A. playing telephones, pounding boards, playing with pots and pans
    B. watching television, finger painting, pounding boards

C. clay molding, playing with pots and pans, doll house
D. playing telephones, finger painting, clay molding (13:59,60,61)

30. Angry feelings in a preschooler, which may result from hospitalization, can be worked off through the use of
    A. pounding boards, puzzles, story books
    B. puzzles, doll houses, clay molding
    C. play injection for the nurse, pounding board, puppet shows
    D. clay molding, play injection for the nurse, pounding boards (13:60,61)

31. What are the purposes of communicating with parents?
    1. provides an opportunity for parents to ventilate their feelings and relieve tension
    2. obtains and transmits information
    3. motivates them in direction of understanding and resolving own problems
    4. acquaints parents with different personality types of members of health team
    A. 1, 2, and 4
    B. 1, 4, and 3
    C. all except 4
    D. all of the above (13:62)

32. Which of the following could *not* be expected of the nurse in relationships with parents and children?
    1. she understands that all behavior is meaningful, although meaning may not always be too clear
    2. she begins to build a working relation with parents and child from her first contact with them, regardless of setting
    3. she should be willing to acknowledge parents' rights to their own decisions concerning their child, even though she may not agree with them
    4. she should work with both parents and child to prevent expression of negative emotions
    A. 1, 2, and 3
    B. 1, 3, and 4
    C. all except 3
    D. all except 4 (13:63,64)

33. Anxiety in parents during a child's illness is most commonly manifested by
    A. restlessness, irritability, trembling, withdrawal, coarse or wavery voice
    B. angry, hostile, aggressive behavior toward nurses and physician caring for their child
    C. extreme dependence on hospital staff for care of child, loss of appetite, reluctance in visiting child, insistence on rooming-in, disregard for ward policies
    D. all except C (13:65)

34. When the nurse detects anxiety in the parent, her first task is to
    A. report her observation to doctor
    B. consult with hospital chaplain or psychiatrist for best approach to make
    C. identify cause(s) of anxiety
    D. none of the above (13:65)

35. If parents blame themselves for their child's illness, the most appropriate thing for the nurse to do is to
    A. convince them that a mistake can be made
    B. explain real cause of illness to them and convey to them her belief that they are competent
    C. give sincere praise for things they have done well to increase their self-confidence
    D. refer them to another helpful professional person (13:65,66)

36. Which of the following factors is likely to magnify parental anxiety about the child's illness and hospitalization?
    A. fear of strange environment in hospital and of unknown
    B. fear that child will suffer and that condition is infectious and may spread to other members of family
    C. fear of unbearable financial obligations
    D. all of the above (13:66)

37. A mother is anxious because only the nurses are giving her child care. Which of the following are appropriate courses of action for the nurse to take?

1. suggest tactfully that mother partially care for child herself
2. explain to her what she can do for and with her child
3. discuss situation in a nursing team conference
4. accept this as natural and identify cause of anxiety
   A. 1, 2 and 3
   B. 1, 3 and 4
   C. 1 and 2
   D. all of the above (13:66)

38. Which of the following is *not* true about illness and hospitalization of children?
   A. hospitalization is not necessarily a traumatic experience for child or adolescent
   B. what hospitalization means to child will depend upon his stage of maturity and past experiences
   C. sensory deprivation of pediatric patient always occurs if child is being cared for in an incubator or intensive care unit
   D. illness can mean pain, restraint of movement, long sleepless periods, and dependence (13:66)

39. Which of the following are basic requirements of pediatric nursing?
   1. great patience and tenderness
   2. strong background in child growth and development
   3. ability to control emotions and prevent personal involvement with patient and family
   4. ability to express emotions in times of stress and still function efficiently
      A. 1, 2 and 4
      B. 1, 2 and 3
      C. 2, 3 and 4
      D. 2 and 4 (13:68,69)

40. When a hospitalized child is found to be provoking fights with other children in the ward, the nurse should
   A. bring about changes in his habits by behavior modification
   B. isolate him in a single bed unit until he learns to play with others
   C. ask his parents to come in for counseling and guidance
   D. condemn act, but not child or teaching of his parents (13:69)

41. The role of the nurse in the admission procedure is primarily
   A. complementary to that of mother and child
   B. equivalent to that of hospital hostess
   C. that of a health educator
   D. that of a health expert (13:71)

42. Ways in which the nurse may make a parent feel more secure and calm in the hospital, and the child less restless include the following, *except*
   A. interviewing parent by another health professional, while nurse takes the child to his unit
   B. introducing herself to mother and child
   C. giving mother a friendly welcome
   D. explaining admission procedure and answering questions clearly (13:71)

43. Which of the following is *not* true about the taking of vital signs of children?
   A. temperature, pulse and respiration should always be taken upon admission
   B. blood pressure is taken only if ordered by the doctor on admission
   C. rectal temperature reading, using either glass or electronic thermometer, should be taken last
   D. to some children, taking of rectal temperature represents a real invasion of their bodies (13:71)

44. Temperature readings may be expressed in either Centigrade or Fahrenheit degrees according to the policy of the agency. A temperature of 104° Fahrenheit is equivalent to how many Centigrade degrees?
   A. 38°
   B. 40°
   C. 39°
   D. 41° (13:71)

45. If the child is to have an operation, he may be terrified at the idea of anesthesia. The following ways are helpful in alleviating a child's anxiety and fear, *except*

A. explaining clearly to him that anaesthesia is a special quiet and safe kind of sleep from which he will wake up
B. allowing him to examine the face mask and play with it
C. informing him that he may take a favorite stuffed toy or doll to operating room with him
D. reinforcing the idea that "little men do not cry." (13:73)

46. Which of the following actions are likely to enhance a parent's sense of guilt over the child's illness?
   1. exploring parent's reasons for reluctance to visit child frequently
   2. explaining to parents why nurse has to do all of the child care during the immediate postoperative period
   3. allowing parents to participate in care of their child under nurse's supervision
   4. arranging for mother to talk with doctor or other professional worker, if mother speaks of needing help which nurse cannot give
   A. 1, 2 and 3
   B. 1, 3 and 4
   C. 1 and 2
   D. all except 3 (13:73)

47. Which one of the following is *not* true about medical aseptic technique?
   A. it is necessary whenever patient and his belongings are contaminated
   B. its purpose is to prevent transmission of bacteria from one child to another, or to personnel who care for him
   C. it is observed as long as it is so specified in doctor's order
   D. it generally excludes nurses with abrasions on their hands (13:76)

48. The destruction of pathogenic organisms carried out continuously while the child is isolated is termed
   A. concurrent disinfection
   B. terminal disinfection
   C. partial disinfection
   D. ad interim disinfection (13:77)

49. Which one of the following is *not* true about the wearing of masks?
   A. if a mask is worn, it should cover both the nose and mouth
   B. a mask should be worn once and then discarded
   C. the use of a wet mask is not necessarily ineffective
   D. a mask worn by a nurse is considered ineffective after one-half hour of use (13:77)

50. Which of the following nursing behaviors would be least likely to stabilize a positive nurse-parent learning situation during a child's hospitalization?
   A. thoroughly explaining admission procedure and answering carefully all questions asked by parent
   B. knowing the level of parents' background of experience and understanding of the child's illness
   C. requiring parent to give basic physical care to hospitalized child
   D. demonstrating how to meet the child's emotional needs while giving physical care (13:70)

51. In planning diversional activity for a 10-year-old boy you must recognize that chilren of this age
   A. need approval from peers
   B. enjoy participating in mixed groups
   C. gain recognition by producing
   D. A and C (13:612)

52. Sue, age 15, was hospitalized for an extended period to correct her orthopedic problem. She developed an attitude of detachment, boredom, and negativism which was probably an attempt to
   A. call attention to her newly developed femininity
   B. mask her anxiety about her illness and future
   C. act out one aspect of adolescent ambivalence
   D. cover up her feelings of inferiority and guilt (13:684,685)

53. Demerol (35 mgm) and Scopolamine (0.24 mgm) are ordered for a preoperative medication. Given an ampule of Scopolamine in which 1 cc = 0.4 mgm, which of the following is appropriate to administer?

A. 5 minims
B. 7 minims
C. 9 minims
D. 11 minims   (4:340)

54. To be able to support a dying child and his parents effectively the nurse should
    1. acquire a deep belief in a deity and a life after death
    2. work out her own personal philosophy concerning the meaning of life and death
    3. discuss with a friend her own distress regarding the child's diagnosis
    4. understand the child's and parents' concept of death
    A. 1 and 2
    B. 2 and 4
    C. 3 and 4
    D. 1 and 3   (13:85)

55. What is the best method for comforting a hospitalized infant who cries frequently for her mother?
    1. give her a favorite toy to hold
    2. move her crib nearer to the corridor
    3. allow mother to stay with her and hold her
    4. stay with her and hold her
    A. 1 and 4
    B. 1 and 3
    C. 2 and 4
    D. 3 and 4   (13:67)

56. Which one of the following is true about crisis?
    A. reorganization levels are always reached following crisis
    B. the crisis does not need to be perceived as such by the family for crisis to occur
    C. unresolved key problems are repressed until after resolution of the crisis
    D. the crisis problem may be either solved, redefined or avoided   (13:62,63)

57. Use of which of the following methods would be best to prepare a five-year-old boy for a planned hospitalization for tonsillectomy?
    A. tell him about his hospitalization just before he is ready to leave for the hospital
    B. tell him he will be going to the hospital where there are lots of toys and other children with whom to play
    C. call the hospital and find out the usual surgical routine and then, a few days before his admission, explain to him very simply about hospitalization
    D. take him to visit a friend who recently had tonsils out, and ask him to tell Tommy all about his experience
                                  (13:556)

58. Which of the following signs should concern you most when taking care of a child who just had a tonsillectomy?
    1. frequent swallowing
    2. vomiting dark red blood
    3. noisy respirations
    4. pulse rate of 140
    5. respiratory rate of 20
    A. 1, 2 and 3
    B. 1, 2 and 5
    C. 1, 3 and 4
    D. 2, 4 and 5   (13:558)

59. Make-believe play provides the hospitalized child with an opportunity to
    A. accept a mother substitute
    B. reject the reality of the hospital
    C. learn to know other children and make friends
    D. cope with his fears and anxieties
                                  (13:535,536)

60. A hospitalized child, age 6, is overprotective of his toys. This is
    A. normal, considering that the child's sense of security has been threatened
    B. normal, since he only understands the concept of ownership
    C. abnormal, as child should share now
    D. abnormal, as child usually pays little attention to toys at this age   (13:66)

61. Anaclitic depression follows which of the following sequence of responses?
    A. protest to denial to despair
    B. denial to protest to despair
    C. denial to despair to protest
    D. protest to despair to denial
                                  (13:451,452)

62. A 3-year-old child, just admitted to the hospital, plays individually in a corner and

avoids other children. How should you respond to this situation?
A. watch child more closely
B. make immediate efforts to involve him in play with others
C. recognize this as a possible response to the stress of hospitalization
D. A and C (13:450,451)

63. Many of the newer regulations in hospital settings are aimed at meeting the emotional as well as physical needs of the child. Which of the following regulations ignores this approach?
A. medical rounds with discussion at the bedside
B. unrestricted visiting hours
C. provision for rooming-in as needed
D. including mother in the admission procedure (13:57)

64. A child is to have blood drawn for diagnostic studies. The nurse feels responsible for explaining the procedure to him but his mother thinks he should not be told. The nurse should
A. concede to the desires of his mother since the final responsibility for him lies with her
B. explain to his mother that he will be more cooperative if he understands the procedure
C. invite the mother to remain with him during the procedure
D. wait until his mother leaves and then explain the procedure to him (13:23)

B. The High-Risk Infant

Directions: This part of the test consists of a situation followed by a series of statements or questions. Study the situation and select the best answer to each statement or question that follows.

Answer items 65 to 71 based on the information given.

65. Mickey Mantle, a 2400 gm premature infant, was admitted to the neonatal intensive care unit following his delivery in severe respiratory distress. Which of the following signs would be seen in Mickey?
A. respiration above 60, intercostal retractions, cyanosis, flaring of nostrils
B. respirations below 10, intercostal retractions, cyanosis, flaring of nostrils
C. respirations at 40 but irregular, absence of retractions, tachycardia, flaring of nostrils
D. irregular respirations, tachycardia, intercostal retractions (13:159,163)

66. Mickey requires assisted ventilation the first 3 days of life. The nurse frequently suctions off his nasotracheal tube. Which of the following is *not* true in relation to suctioning Mickey?
A. suction is applied when entering the tube and released when removing the tube
B. the procedure should be done rapidly to prevent bradycardia
C. the oral pharynx need not be suctioned when a nasotracheal tube is in place
D. suctioning should be done following each feeding (13:161)

67. Mickey's parents were very traumatized when they first saw their tiny baby and the equipment surrounding him. The nurse's best response to lessen their fear and enable them to relate to the baby should be to
A. explain the equipment to them and assure them how fortunate they are to have their child in such a scientific place
B. show them a sicker baby so that Mickey won't look as sick in comparison
C. explain the equipment simply and have them wash their hands and give them the opportunity to touch the baby
D. have them wash their hands and insist they touch the baby so their fear will be removed (13:162,163)

68. Vitamin K is administered intramuscularly to Mickey to
A. prepare him for blood loss
B. aid in the clotting process
C. prevent destruction of red blood cells
D. prevent infection (13:161)

69. Retrolental fibroplasia is a disease which occurs most frequently in small premature infants. Its cause is generally attributed to
    A. transitory hypoxia
    B. oxygen toxicity
    C. drug addiction
    D. toxemia of pregnancy   (28:249)

70. Mickey was placed in the incubator. The nurse regulates the temperature in the incubator on the basis of the temperature of
    A. the environment
    B. his extremities
    C. his body
    D. 88° F is set for all premature infants   (13:163)

71. Mickey was fed initially by gavage by the nurse. His mother expressed fear and anger upon seeing this because her physician said that the baby was doing fine. The nurse's best response should be
    A. "This method will prevent infection of his mouth with a rubber nipple. Your baby has a low resistance to infection making this necessary."
    B. "Your baby could vomit and inhale his formula if we use a bottle."
    C. "It is very busy today and this is the only way I can quickly and safely feed your baby."
    D. "Your baby is continuing to do well, but it tires him and uses energy (calories) when he sucks on the nipple."   (13:163)

Directions: For each of the following multiple choice questions, select the ONE most appropriate answer.

72. Baby Jamison, a premature weighing 3.5 lbs., was immediately put into an incubator which was warmed to a temperature of 99° F. The nurse's rationale supporting this action is that
    A. prematures metabolize at such an increased rate that their temperature must be maintained at a higher level than 98.6
    B. prematures have limited ability to regulate their own temperature
    C. the acidosis in the premature resulting from labor and delivery decreases the infant's temperature
    D. the decreased amounts of surfactant produced by the infant affects his ability to regulate his temperature   (28:248)

73. Which of the following is a complication due to the administration of a high percentage of oxygen to the newborn and/or premature?
    A. retrolental fibroplasia
    B. central nervous system depression
    C. polycythemia
    D. metabolic acidosis   (7:146)

74. Which of the following is the single most important mode of control of nursery infections due to staphylococci?
    A. antibiotic administration to all premature infants
    B. use of gloves and masks
    C. strict handwashing techniques
    D. exclusion of everyone but nursing and medical personnel from the nursery   (28:252)

75. Baby Robertson, a 2.8 lb. premature infant, showed signs of jaundice at age 2 days. He has no blood incompatibility or liver disease. Which of the following is the best explanation for this physiological phenomenon?
    A. increased level of water-solubles, conjugated bilirubin in blood stream
    B. high concentration of fetal hemoglobin at birth
    C. decreased activity of glucuronyl transferase especially in premature infants
    D. decreased erythropoietic processes during premature's initial few weeks of life   (7:153,154)

76. As part of the treatment for his hyperbilirubinemia, Baby Robertson was placed under the phototherapy light with his eyes protected by a shield. The nurse as a result must be aware of which of the following problems?
    A. elevated temperature due to heat from light

B. need for tactile and visual stimulation
C. lethargy because of infant's isolation
D. possible nausea and vomiting as a result of increased absorption of ultraviolet light (7:155)

77. Which of the following is the most important nutrient for all infants during their first hours of life?
A. protein
B. minerals
C. carbohydrates
D. vitamins (7:159)

78. Which of the following is the *most* important factor affecting the parents' ability to give adequate care to their high-risk infant?
A. extent of maternal-child separation
B. guilt feelings in the mother
C. cultural attitudes toward birth of an unhealthy infant
D. length of time spent by infant in an incubator (7:161,162)

79. Baby Jones, a premature infant, with a weak sucking reflex, has been fed via gavage. The nurse, in deciding whether to intubate through the nasopharynx or oropharynx, should be aware of which of the following?
A. passage of the tube down esophagus can cause bradycardia
B. infants are obligatory nose breathers
C. premature infants have extremely sensitive gag reflexes
D. frequent passage of gavage tubing may irritate mucous membranes (7:159)

80. Which of the following must be taken into consideration in supplying the diet for the premature infant?
A. larger volumes must be given to supply their increased need for calories and fluids
B. greater formula concentrations are required to provide increased need for calories without overhydration
C. lesser formula concentrations are given as the premature has lesser caloric needs while still meeting his fluid needs
D. smaller volume of regular formula concentrate is provided because child has limited gastrointestinal capacity (28:253)

81. Which of the following classifications of newborns has the highest mortality rate?
A. immature 20-27 wks.
B. premature
C. preterm
D. post-mature (7:139)

82. Which of the following infants could be classified as premature by gestational age?
1. Boy Jones, weight 10.5 lbs., son of a diabetic mother
2. Girl Smith, weight 3.6 lbs., daughter of a mother with incompetency of the cervix
3. Boy Campbell, weight 3 lbs., gestational age 39 weeks, son of a mother without prenatal care
4. Boy Porter, weight 4.5 lbs., gestational age 43 weeks, suffered meconium aspiration in utero
A. 1 and 3
B. 2 and 4
C. 1 and 2
D. 3 and 4 (7:140)

83. Which of the following are characteristics of the premature which may predispose the infant to illness?
1. thin and delicate mucous membranes
2. increased production of surfactant
3. overactivity of the liver and spleen
4. loss of fluid to a greater percent than older infants
5. fragile capillary structures
A. 2, 3 and 4
B. 1, 4 and 5
C. 1, 2 and 5
D. all of the above (7:141-42)

84. The most common abnormal finding among premature babies is
A. cerebral palsy
B. retrolental fibroplasia
C. perceptual-motor difficulties
D. severe deafness (10:317)

Situational Problems

85. When there is evidence of a significant disruption in family cohesiveness and deterioration of marital and parent-sibling relations, the role of the nurse is primarily to
    A. advise parents to seek psychiatric consultation
    B. hire a visiting nurse
    C. assist parents to mobilize their resources
    D. all of the above (10:323)

86. In which of the following areas do mothers of premature babies particularly need help?
    A. avoidance of overprotection of child
    B. shunning away from socialization
    C. financial obligation
    D. family planning (10:323)

87. Which of the following measures is *least* effective in handling spitting up problems following feeding of a premature infant?
    A. propping him up after feeding
    B. frequent bubbling during feeding
    C. slowed feedings
    D. lying flat on back during feeding (10:328)

88. In the first year of life, aggressive behavior is closely linked to
    A. oral activity
    B. anal activity
    C. genital activity
    D. genito-anal activity (10:329)

C. Accidents

Directions: This part of the test consists of a situation followed by a series of statements or questions. Study the situation and select the best answer to each statement or question that follows.

Timmy Gordon, a 2-year-old child, is seen in the emergency room. His mother found him with the empty bottle of baby aspirin. She thinks there were 10 aspirin tablets in the bottle. She brought him to the emergency room at once. She had found the empty bottle 20 minutes before.

Answer items 89–99 based on the information given.

89. Since Timmy's mother acted so promptly, you would look for which of the following signs as the *first* sign of aspirin poisoning?
    A. vomiting
    B. drowsiness
    C. hyperpnea
    D. convulsion (13:473)

90. Since the salicylates inhibit the formation of prothrombin by the liver, which of the following conditions might be observed in Timmy if immediate treatment were not instituted?
    A. hyperpyrexia
    B. purpura
    C. vomiting
    D. sweating (13:473)

91. Immediate treatment for Timmy would likely include
    A. lavage
    B. administration of syrup of ipecac
    C. parenteral fluids
    D. all of the above (13:473)

92. Children this age commonly ingest drugs because they
    A. have great curiosities
    B. put almost everything in their mouths
    C. are good eaters and will eat anything
    D. A and B (13:417,418)

93. Mrs. Gordon seems concerned about his behavior. She describes Timmy as not being interested in playing with other children. "He doesn't fight with them, but simply ignores them and plays by himself in the same room." Your *best* response would be
    A. "As long as they don't fight, don't worry about it."
    B. "It's not unusual for children this age to fight, be happy that's no problem."
    C. "Toddlers seldom play with other children, but enjoy playing in the same room."
    D. "Children this age are inconsistent in play patterns, don't worry about it." (13:436)

94. Timmy had been treated for pinworms six months ago. His mother has noticed some

redness around the anus when bathing Timmy. She asks you, "Could he have pinworms again?" Your *best* response should be
A. "Yes, it's possible; let's do the scotch tape test right now."
B. "No, the treatment prescribed before is effective for at least 1 year."
C. "Yes, it's possible; he'd better have a rectal swab done while he is here."
D. "Yes, it's possible; using scotch tape, press around the anal area when he is asleep." (13:468)

95. Mrs. Gordon asks you if her two other children, ages 4 and 6, are likely to have pinworms. Your *best* response would be
A. "No, pinworm infestation affects only the toddlers."
B. "Probably, since children are susceptible and this condition is frequent when children are in close contact with somebody who is infested."
C. "I really can't tell you. I'll refer you to the doctor."
D. "You are concerned about Timmy's condition; I understand." (13:467)

96. Now Timmy's mother asks you how she might recognize possible pinworm infestation in her daughter. You should tell her that she is most likely to observe in her daughter
A. vomiting, colic, urticaria, itching about anus in daytime and night
B. anorexia, mild fever, lethargy
C. poor appetite, weight loss, irritability, itching about anus at night
D. sleeplessness, anorexia, nausea, pruritus ani (13:467,469)

97. Mrs. Gordon would like to know how to prevent reinfestation. Which of the following instructions is irrelevant?
A. hand hygiene should be strictly carried out especially in mornings and before meals
B. toilet seat should be scrubbed daily
C. bedpan should be cleansed and sterilized after use

D. nails should be cut as short as possible (13:469)

98. Which of the following precautions should you ask Mrs. Gordon to observe at home on the basis of Timmy's accidental ingestion of aspirin?
A. all dangerous substances should be kept out of children's reach, on a high shelf or in a locked cupboard
B. all drugs, household chemicals, and poisons should be kept in tightly closed containers
C. if another toxic ingestion occurs, induce vomiting by giving child glass of milk or water containing salt
D. all of the above (13:472)

99. Which of the following substances would contraindicate the inducement of vomiting following its ingestion?
A. petroleum distillate
B. lye
C. phenobarbital
D. A and B (13:473)

Directions: For each of the following multiple choice questions, select the ONE most appropriate answer.

100. Which of the following is *not* among the five leading causes of death in childhood and adolescence?
A. cardiovascular-renal diseases
B. malignant neoplasms
C. communicable diseases
D. congenital malformations (29:18)

101. Deaths among children and young adults is primarily associated with
A. malignant neoplasms
B. accidents
C. homicides
D. cardiovascular-renal conditions (29:18)

102. Which one of the following does *not* accurately reflect reported findings on accidents?
A. motor vehicle fatalities account for two-fifths of accidental deaths at school age
B. girls are the more frequent victims of drowning than boys

Situational Problems 153

C. fatal accidents among school-age children occur predominantly in recreational and outdoor places
D. types of accidents vary with age, sex, socioeconomic condition, geography, season, and even the time of day (29:19)

103. At about what age do most deaths of bicyclists occur because of collisions with motor vehicles?
 A. 8–12 years
 B. 10–14 years
 C. 12–16 years
 D. 14–18 years (27:19)

D. Burns

Directions: This part of the test consists of a situation followed by a series of statements or questions. Study the situation and select the best answer to each statement or question that follows.

Two-year-old Jerry Ryan was brought to the emergency room of the hospital for treatment of burns on his chest, abdomen, left arm and left leg after he had spilled a pot of hot coffee on himself. The doctor describes the burns as both second and third degree, covering twenty percent of his body.

Answer items 104–109 based on the information given.

104. Which of the following would describe Jerry's second degree burns?
 A. destruction of the epidermis only
 B. destruction of the epidermis with severe pain
 C. destruction of epidermis and dermis with pain
 D. destruction of epidermis, dermis, and nerve endings (13:475)

105. An eschar is best defined as
 A. thickened, roughened line of skin that is elevated above surrounding tissue
 B. tough coagulum of necrotic tissue that develops over heat injured area
 C. an aggregation of suppurative material derived from tissue debridement
 D. a band of scar tissue that causes deformity by contraction (13:475)

106. The most effective way to prevent contractures from forming in Jerry's arm and leg is to
 A. maintain body alignment
 B. establish routine passive exercise for him
 C. turn him from side to side
 D. bathe him in Hubbard tank twice a day (13:480)

107. Because burns place undue stress on the body, after the first 48 hours the nurse must be alert for
 A. headache and convulsions as a result of generalized toxicity
 B. labored respirations due to pulmonary congestion
 C. gastrointestinal bleeding from a Curling's ulcer (abd. discomfort)
 D. weakness and fatigue due to decreased adrenal functioning (13:478)

108. Jerry screams during the dressing change. The nurse should
 A. try to quiet Jerry and tell him, "It will soon be finished."
 B. ask the doctor to do the dressing change when his mother is there to comfort him
 C. tell Jerry, "It's all right to cry. I know this hurts."
 D. try to calm Jerry and tell him, "We have to change your dressing." (13:450)

109. After the dressing change the nurse should
 A. hold and rock Jerry to convey that the nurse cares about him
 B. return him to his room and leave him so he can rest after an exhausting procedure
 C. distract him with a game so he will forget about the pain
 D. give him a puppet which will stimulate him to talk (13:455)

Bobby, a five-year-old, is being admitted for plastic surgery for repair of scars resulting from burns. Two years ago he had been a patient for six months when he pulled a pan of hot fat off the stove and was severely burned on his abdomen and both thighs. He has had extensive grafting in this area and some contractures have developed. During the admission procedure, Bobby clings to his mother and appears shy.

Answer items 110–117 based on the information given.

110. Understanding the stages in personality development, you would exercise the *greatest* amount of care and persuasion when you
    A. measure his height and weight
    B. take his temperature (rectally)
    C. introduce him to his roommates
    D. make the nursing assessment, examine the scars to describe them (13:549)

111. Bobby's mother says he's been soiling his pants occasionally during the past two weeks, "ever since our last visit to the doctor." She asks, "Is this normal?" Which of the following statements would be the best response?
    A. "It may be a sign of an intestinal disorder, the doctor will be alerted."
    B. "It is probably a passing phase and he will forget about it in time."
    C. "He is probably concerned about what will happen to him; he needs your love and support."
    D. "It's normal for children to go back to former behavior when they are frightened; don't worry." (13:549)

112. Which of the following might *enhance* the stress of hospitalization for Bobby?
    A. encouraging his mother to spend as much time as possible with him
    B. asking to be assigned to Bobby on a continuous basis
    C. providing Bobby with puppets and encouraging him to express himself
    D. placing Bobby in the same unit as the school-aged boys to encourage him to play (13:533)

113. When Bobby's mother leaves, he screams and kicks and begs her not to go. The *best* action is to
    A. distract him by taking him to the playroom to play
    B. point out that he is a "big boy" and must not cry
    C. listen to his feelings and reassure him that his mother will return
    D. point out that another boy's mother left and he isn't crying (13:543)

114. You are attempting to gain Bobby's trust. Which of the following techniques should you use?
    A. maintain a calm, patient manner
    B. plan his activities to keep him busy
    C. respect his need to regress
    D. all of the above (13:549,550)

115. Which of the following is true concerning children of Bobby's age? They
    A. believe that hospitalization is punishment
    B. engage in symbolic play with great imagination
    C. react well to making choices between actions
    D. are very inquisitive and ask many questions (13:549)

116. You are preparing Bobby for surgery. Which of the following statements would be *most* reassuring to a child of this age?
    A. "You will not die, so concentrate on how much better you will feel when it is over."
    B. "Only yours legs will be operated on; they will not operate on your head, your arms, or your body."
    C. "You will go to sleep and when you wake up your mommy and daddy will be here."
    D. "Your legs will have bandages on them when you awake but there will be no bleeding." (13:549)

117. In an effort to reduce the stress of hospitalization for Bobby, you might
    A. encourage his mother to spend as much time as possible with him
    B. ask to be assigned to Bobby on a continuous basis

C. provide Bobby with puppets and encourage him to express himself
D. all of the above (13:549,550)

Susy, a 3-year-old, was severely burned when she pulled a pot of boiling water off the stove. She has second and third degree burns of the anterior chest (¼ of trunk) and the anterior surfaces of both arms and thighs.

Answer items 118 through 122 based on the information given.

118. If you had been present at the time of the accident, which first aid treatment would have been the most appropriate?
    A. apply cold water and cover with a clean dressing
    B. liberally apply any salt-free cooking oil
    C. liberally apply a salve
    D. cover with a sterile dressing only (13:476)

119. Electrolytes as well as fluids are lost from extensively burned areas. The following are signs of metabolic acidosis *except*
    A. Kussmaul respirations
    B. depressed level of consciousness and dull headache
    C. glucose loss in urine with increased flow
    D. glucose retention with decreased flow of urine (13:476)

120. In caring for Susy in the first 24 hours, you should
    A. carefully regulate I.V. flow and watch for signs of respiratory distress
    B. record vital signs, looking for signs of hypervolemic shock
    C. observe level of consciousness and urinary flow
    D. all of the above (13:476)

121. When Susy progresses to the point where she can take solid foods, the diet which would be best suited for her is
    A. high caloric, high protein
    B. high caloric, normal protein
    C. high caloric, low residue
    D. normal diet with forced fluids (13:476)

122. In caring for Susy, which of the following measures would be *most* supportive?
    A. place Susy in a bright room with pictures and other toddlers
    B. allow mother to spend as much time as possible with Susy
    C. conserve her energy by feeding her and encouraging quiet play
    D. spend as much time with Susy as possible, reading and playing quiet games (13:480)

E. Fractures

Directions: This part of the test consists of a situation followed by a series of statements or questions. Study the situation and select the best answer to each statement or question that follows.

You are assigned to care for Jim, a 10-year-old, who is in traction with a fractured femur. The fracture was sustained in an automobile accident in which his father was seriously injured. Jim is anxiously awaiting the day he is put into a cast. Mr. Todd, his teacher, the driver of the car, escaped without injury and comes in to see him each day.

Answer items 123 through 131 based on the information given.

123. Which of the following activities would be *most* suitable for Jim?
    A. dramatizing with puppets
    B. building with popsicle sticks
    C. modeling with play dough
    D. watching television (13:612)

124. When asked about how he broke his leg, Jim replies, "In an automobile accident, but it wasn't Mr. Todd's fault. He is the best driver there is." You recognize this response as a means of expressing
    A. repression
    B. regression
    C. hero worship
    D. B and C (13:612)

125. If you had a choice in placing Jim in a room *best* suited for him, you would place him in a room

A. with another 10-year-old and a 5-year-old since Jim has a 5-year-old brother
B. with two other 10-year-olds who are ambulatory and can move about freely
C. by himself, since boys this age are sensitive about body image
D. with another 10-year-old who is also confined to bed (13:612)

126. You notice that Jim seems careless and disinterested in brushing his teeth, combing his hair, etc. His 12-year-old roommate exhibits the same behavior. Your *best* response is to
A. use this as an opportunity to do some health teaching
B. use his interest in the opposite sex to encourage good grooming
C. encourage good grooming but don't dwell on it
D. appeal to Jim's mother to work with him since he loves her (13:612)

127. According to Erikson's theory of personality development, Jim's core problem is
A. industry vs. inferiority
B. autonomy vs. shame
C. initiative vs. guilt
D. trust vs. mistrust (13:601)

128. You know that the signs and symptoms that Jim might present if he were not treated properly would include the following, *except*
A. inability to bear weight
B. pain on movement
C. local tenderness
D. asymmetry of shoulders (13:481)

129. On the basis of the treatment instituted on Jim, his fracture should be of what type?
A. greenstick
B. compound
C. simple
D. incomplete (13:481)

130. The traction apparatus commonly used for children having a fractured femur is Bryant's traction, and the method is by
A. horizontal suspension
B. vertical suspension
C. weight suspension
D. pulley suspension (13:481)

131. Which of the following would *not* be a sign that Jim's cast had been applied too tightly?
A. pallor, discoloration or cyanosis of skin
B. edema of toes
C. warm, dry toes
D. loss of sensation (13:482)

F. Leukemia

Directions: This part of the test consists of a situation followed by a series of statements or questions. Study the situation and select the best answer to each statement or question that follows.

You are caring for Susan White, a 5-year-old girl with leukemia. Her temperature is 104°F. She is extremely irritable and is bleeding from the gums.

Answer items 132 through 146 based on the information given.

132. In addition to the aforenoted clinical signs, which of the following manifestations would you expect to show?
1. pallor
2. thrombi
3. abdominal pain
4. enlarged lymph nodes
5. diarrhea
A. 1, 2 and 5
B. 1, 3 and 4
C. 2, 3 and 5
D. 3, 4 and 5 (13:573)

133. In developing a nursing care plan for Susan you would include
1. oral hygiene four times a day
2. gentle handling of the extremities
3. small, frequent feedings
4. a quiet, but pleasant atmosphere
5. frequent change in position
A. 1, 2 and 3
B. 1, 3 and 4
C. 2, 4 and 5
D. all of the above (13:516,577)

134. Which of the following findings would *not* be expected in Susan's blood count?
    A. white blood cells—5,000/cu. mm.
    B. red blood cells—2.5 million/cu. mm.
    C. hemoglobin—6 gm/100 ml.
    D. platelet count—350,000/cu. mm.
    (13:572)

135. The main reason children with leukemia have trouble with bleeding is that
    A. their white blood cells are short lived, not mature
    B. tissue destruction interferes with platelet production
    C. anemia causes blood to flow faster with more pressure on capillary walls
    D. poor appetite results in lack of maturation factors for cell production
    (13:572)

136. In preparing Susan for a bone marrow aspiration, which of the following is the best first approach by the nurse?
    A. simple explanation of the procedure to be done
    B. allow child some measure of control during the procedure
    C. approve of her efforts toward control of her body
    D. permit expression of feelings about the procedure
    (13:577)

A remission was effected for 15 months. Her relapse was then treated on an outpatient basis by changing her medication to Methotrexate. She remained asymptomatic for another 3 months and then complained of headaches, nausea and vomiting. It was subsequently necessary to admit her to the hospital.

137. Susan was treated as an outpatient for as long as possible to
    A. provide more time to prepare her for hospitalization
    B. involve her mother in her care
    C. permit Susan to live as normal a life as possible
    D. minimize the cost of her lengthy, terminal illness
    (13:576)

138. When Mrs. White reached Susan's room on admission, she began to cry and walked away. You are the nurse admitting Susan. Your *best* initial approach would be
    A. "I'll be right back, I need to show your mother where the lounge is."
    B. Take Susan's hand and say, "You probably feel uncomfortable and frightened; if I am right, just squeeze my hand."
    C. "Have you ever been in the hospital before, Susan?"
    D. "I am (insert your first name), and I will be your nurse until 3:00."
    (13:576,577)

139. The nurse should observe and record the side effects of any drugs used. Which of the following precautions should be observed when *vicristine* is used?
    A. utilize a footboard
    B. relieve constipation
    C. prepare child for possible alopecia
    D. all of the above
    (13:577)

140. The immediate nursing goal when caring for a hemophiliac following a bleeding episode is to
    A. prevent external trauma
    B. control capillary bleeding
    C. give medication to relax the patient
    D. keep the patient quiet and rested
    (13:576)

141. The most important nursing concern in caring for a leukemic child with severe anemia is to
    A. teach proper diet to mother
    B. conserve child's energy
    C. protect her from infection
    D. observe for respiratory distress
    (13:576)

142. A common complication following bleeding episodes in children with hemophilia is
    A. thrombocytopenia
    B. hemarthrosis
    C. hemangioma
    D. aseptic necrosis
    (13:578,579)

143. The nurse can be of substantial help to Susan and her family during the terminal

phase of the child's illness by demonstrating the following, *except*
A. accepting parents' way of expressing fear and grief
B. keeping Susan's nose and throat clean, and her lips and mouth moist
C. leaving parents alone at her bedside when Susan lapses into unconsciousness
D. allowing parents to participate in Susan's basic care (13:577,578)

144. The normal white blood cell count is
A. 12,000–17,000/cu. mm.
B. 8,000–13,000/cu. mm.
C. 5,000–10,000/cu. mm.
D. 40,000–50,000/cu. mm. (13:572)

145. The most common immediate cause of death in leukemia is
A. intracranial hemorrhage
B. intercurrent infection
C. myocardial infarction
D. pulmonary embolism (13:573)

146. Which of the following is *not* true concerning leukemia?
A. it is a malignant neoplasm involving all blood-forming organs
B. its cause is unknown
C. cure is presently known and treatment is specific
D. more than 50% of cases of leukemia in children occur below five years of age (13:572,573,574)

G. Rheumatic Fever

Directions: This part of the test consists of a situation followed by a series of statements or questions. Study the situation and select the best answer to each statement or question that follows.

Billy Love, age 10, complained of a sore throat three weeks ago. Now he has a temperature of 101° F, pulse 136, respiration 24, blood pressure 110/80 mm Hg. Although his ankles, knees, and wrists are not swollen, Billy has some tenderness in these areas upon examination.

Answer items 147 through 161 based on the information given.

147. The doctor made the diagnosis of rheumatic fever and has ordered complete bedrest. In order to assist in realizing the primary goals of Billy's care, the nurse should plan to
A. continuously attend him, thereby having opportunities for good observation
B. have different members of the nursing team with him at staggered intervals so that he may be closely observed
C. provide long periods of uninterrupted rest during which he is not disturbed for care
D. turn the responsibility for self-care over to Billy as rapidly as possible so that he doesn't become dependent (13:647)

148. An antistreptolysin-o-titer of 625 indicates that he has
A. few body defenses against streptococci
B. acquired immunity to streptococcal toxins
C. recently had a streptococcal infection
D. never been exposed to streptococci (13:644,645)

149. It is the nurse's responsibility to observe Billy closely for which of the following clinical symptoms of rheumatic fever?
A. diarrhea and urinary incontinence
B. subcutaneous nodules and choreiform movements
C. vesicular rash and chest pain
D. nausea and vomiting (13:645)

150. In an effort to keep a child with rheumatic fever comfortable and minimize joint discomfort the nurse should
A. exercise the involved joints for ten minutes three times a day
B. apply analgesic ointment and massage the joints gently
C. apply warm soaks to his joints throughout the acute phase of his illness
D. support the joints using sand bags, rolls, pillows (13:647)

151. Billy is placed on large doses of aspirin. The nurse caring for him should know that toxic effects of acetylsalicylic acid include
    1. headache
    2. diarrhea
    3. tinnitus
    4. purpura
    5. hypoventilation
    6. elevated blood pressure
    A. 1, 2 and 6
    B. 1, 3 and 4
    C. 2, 4 and 5
    D. 3, 5 and 6 (13:473)

152. Major criteria of rheumatic fever are
    A. migratory polyarthritis and carditis
    B. carditis and chorea
    C. carditis and subcutaneous nodules
    D. spontaneous nosebleeds and joint pain (13:645)

153. Which of the following is of *least* importance in understanding rheumatic fever?
    A. carditis often leads to permanent heart damage
    B. bedrest is important to minimize scarring
    C. pain adds to stress of immobilization
    D. first attack may not be observed at all (13:645)

154. Which of the following activities would be best for an 11-year-old girl with acute rheumatic fever, assuming she is interested in each?
    A. flashlight tag and pillow fight
    B. painting murals and weaving potholders
    C. ring toss and carving soap
    D. making jewelry and discussions (13:649,659)

155. The seriousness of repeated recurrences of rheumatic fever lies in
    A. progressive degeneration of the central nervous system
    B. permanently deformed joints
    C. chronic valvular disease
    D. presence of chronic infections which are resistant to therapy (13:651)

156. The *most* suitable activities for Billy which you should encourage during the convalescent period include
    1. making model airplanes
    2. doing his school work
    3. playing quiet games in the playroom
    4. watching television
    5. reading comic books
    A. 1, 2 and 3
    B. 1, 3 and 4
    C. 1, 4 and 5
    D. 2, 4 and 5 (13:649)

157. As a public health nurse you make a visit to evaluate the home situation before Billy's discharge. Which of the following conditions should concern you *most*?
    A. there is no hot water in the home
    B. Billy will sleep in the same room as his brother Joe, who has chronic tonsillitis
    C. family lives in a second floor walk-up apartment
    D. family shares a bathroom with another family on the second floor (13:651)

158. Several weeks after discharge you meet Billy's mother downtown. She complains that Billy is still on bedrest and is very demanding and difficult to manage. Which of the following would be the *best* reply to her?
    A. "We were afraid this would happen. Would you like me to tell Dr. Jones about it?"
    B. "You will just have to be very firm with Billy and he'll get over it."
    C. "These must be very difficult times for both you and your family."
    D. "I'll be happy to tell another public health nurse to stop in to see you." (13:650)

159. Nine months later Billy is readmitted with rheumatic fever occurring with signs of Sydenham's chorea. Signs of Sydenham's chorea are
    A. orthopnea, cyanosis, pain
    B. emotional instability, purposeless movements

C. swollen ankles, elevated temperature
D. "growing pains" and spontaneous nose-bleeds (13:652)

160. The nursing care goal for Billy at this time should be focused on
    A. bedrest
    B. minimal stimulation
    C. administration of anti-inflammatory agents
    D. active and passive exercising (13:652)

161. Sydenham's chorea is otherwise known as
    A. Still's disease
    B. Kahn's disease
    C. Hansen's dance
    D. St. Vitus dance (13:651)

H. Congenital Heart Diseases

Directions: For each of the following multiple choice questions, select the ONE most appropriate answer.

162. Which of the following is *not true* about congenital heart diseases?
    A. most pediatric patients with congenital heart disease are asymptomatic unless they are blue or in cardiac failure
    B. an infant or young child with heart disease sets his or her own pace and does not require parental curtailment of ordinary activity
    C. bacterial endocarditis is a potential risk throughout the lifetime of the person with congenital heart disease
    D. occurrence of cardiac failure is common after the age of six months (23:20)

163. The following patients with congenital heart disease need immediate referral, *except*
    A. cyanotic newborn
    B. child with organic murmur
    C. tachypneic newborn
    D. cyanotic child with unexplained fever (23:15)

164. The first step in the diagnosis of cardiac anomalies is

A. cardiac catheterization
B. angiocardiography
C. determination of presence or absence of cyanosis
D. palpation of peripheral pulses simultaneously in both arms and in an arm and leg (23:11)

165. Which of the following techniques of physical examination may pinpoint a cardiac lesion?
    A. inspection
    B. palpation
    C. percussion
    D. auscultation (23:12)

166. Which of the following is *not* seen in congenital heart disease of the newborn?
    A. tachycardia
    B. pink color
    C. clubbing
    D. weakness (13:231)

167. What symptoms would you expect in a child with patent ductus arteriosus?
    A. he gets slightly blue if he exerts himself a great deal
    B. he has never been blue but he gets shortness of breath if he runs a lot
    C. he squats a great deal of the time
    D. he has great difficulty in eating (13:234)

168. The first signs of cardiac arrest following a cardiac operation are
    A. irregular pulse rate, low blood pressure
    B. edema of ankles, rapid increase in weight
    C. disturbance of sleep during the night, no apparent edema
    D. productive coughing, dyspnea (13:241)

169. You would expect a child with tetralogy of Fallot to have
    A. skin with bluish tint, favoring squatting position
    B. skin with natural pink color and clubbing of fingers and toes
    C. passive tendencies, and to be well behaved

D. retarded growth, but usually normal in intelligence (13:237)

170. Which of the following drugs is most likely to be ordered by the doctor for rapid digitalization and for maintenance therapy?
 A. digitoxin
 B. digoxin
 C. serpasil
 D. Ritalin (23:80)

171. A positive feature of digitoxin is that
 A. its relatively rapid excretion may be useful in dealing with toxicity
 B. its slower excretion rate may lead to a greater stability in myocardial concentration
 C. its rate of excretion depends on glomerular filtration and there is no marked tabular reabsorption of the drug
 D. B and C (23:80)

172. Which of the following signs and symptoms of digitoxin toxicity is most frequently seen in infants and small children?
 A. vomiting
 B. arrhythmias
 C. diarrhea
 D. anorexia (23:77)

You are assigned to care for Jane McHugh, a four-year-old child with the diagnosis of tetralogy of Fallot. The diagnosis was made shortly after birth and she is admitted now for surgery.

173. Clinical manifestations which you would expect Jane to exhibit are
 1. decreased growth rate
 2. exertional dyspnea
 3. fatigue
 4. cyanosis
 5. clubbing of the extremities
 A. 1, 2 and 3
 B. 1, 4 and 5
 C. 2, 3 and 4
 D. all of the above (13:236)

174. A cardiac catheterization is done to determine
 A. location and severity of murmur
 B. the presence of hypertrophy or abnormal configurations
 C. degree and pressure of oxygen in chambers
 D. B and C (13:232)

175. Nursing priorities in caring for a child after a cardiac catheterization using the femoral vein include
 A. elevation of unaffected leg
 B. checking the toes for flushing, fever
 C. application of cold to the cutdown area
 D. checking and comparison of pedal pulses (13:232)

176. Which of the following groups of congenital heart diseases may result in circulation of poorly oxygenated blood through the arteries and veins?
 A. subaortic stenosis, tetralogy of Fallot, transposition of the great vessels
 B. subaortic stenosis, patent ductus arteriosus, coarctation of the aorta
 C. tetralogy of Fallot, complete transposition of the great vessels, atrial septal defect
 D. coarctation of the aorta, patent ductus arteriosus, atrial septal defect (13:232,233,234)

177. A large pulse pressure, dyspnea upon exertion, and retardation in growth are symptoms of
 A. patent ductus arteriosus
 B. coarctation of the aorta
 C. aortic stenosis
 D. pulmonary stenosis (13:234)

178. Following cardiac surgery, Jane has chest drainage. While caring for her in the immediate postoperative period you examine the chest drainage system and expect to find which of the following?
 1. short tubing to restrict Jane's movement in bed
 2. clamps available at the bedside, for emergency use
 3. the fluid level in the tubing has stabilized
 4. bottles are below chest level

5. the amount of drainage from the pleural cavity is recorded regularly on the bottle
   A. 1, 2 and 3
   B. 1, 2 and 4
   C. 2, 4 and 5
   D. 3, 4 and 5   (13:241,242)

179. In the postoperative care of a child who has had cardiac surgery, coughing is of extreme importance. In carrying out this measure the nurse should
   A. encourage coughing every four hours after child has received pain medication
   B. support child's chest firmly with both hands and encourage child to take deep breaths and cough
   C. support child by putting one hand behind the child's back and encourage child to cough
   D. discourage coughing for the first 24 hours while child is having a great deal of pain and then have child cough every two hours   (13:242)

180. Which of the following is true and must be understood about the postoperative care of a patient having chest drainage via gravity through a thoracotomy tube?
   A. bubbling in the drainage bottle indicates that the chest is draining adequately
   B. the fluid in the tubing oscillates between respirations
   C. a greater pressure in the lungs as compared to the pleural space will cause pneumothorax
   D. the *first* important step for the nurse to do, if pneumothorax occurs, is to clamp the thoracotomy tubing   (13:242)

181. Which of the following does *not* relate to the possible home regimen of a child following corrective heart surgery?
   A. conservation of energy
   B. support for mothering figure
   C. provision of activities for acting out increased levels of aggression
   D. resumption of normal diet replacing salt-free diet   (13:242)

182. Which of the following is true concerning congestive heart failure?
   A. it reflects the compensatory measures made by the heart when under physiologic strain or when damaged
   B. fluids move from tissues into the circulatory system
   C. high Fowler's position can help to alleviate pulmonary congestion
   D. inspiratory wheeze may be indicative of congestive heart failure   (13:243)

I. Respiratory Disorders

Directions: This part of the test consists of a situation followed by a series of statements or questions. Study the situation and select the best answer to each statement or question that follows.

Mary Lou Santos, 13-months-old, is admitted to the fourth floor in marked respiratory distress. Her respirations are rapid and labored and her color is dusky. The diagnosis of bronchiolitis is made.

Answer items 183 through 196 based on the information given.

183. The pathophysiological cause of bronchiolitis is a
   A. blockage of air within the air sacs
   B. consolidation of a lobe of the lung
   C. spasm of the smooth muscle of the respiratory tract
   D. congenital malformation which causes repeated respiratory infections   (13:331)

184. Which of the following signs and symptoms would be indicative of laryngotracheobronchitis?
   A. retractions and inspiratory stridor
   B. flaring of the nostrils and expiratory stridor
   C. gradual onset and elevated temperature
   D. A and C   (13:459)

185. Mary Lou frequently cries for her mother. What measures should be taken to comfort her?
   1. give her a favorite toy to hold
   2. move her crib nearer the corridor
   3. allow mother to stay with her and hold her

4. stay with her and hold her
   A. 1 and 4
   B. 1 and 3
   C. 2 and 4
   D. 3 and 4   (13:464)

186. Every time Mary Lou's mother goes home, the child cuddles her teddy bear and refuses to play or respond to the volunteer. You recognize this as
   A. evidence of her insecurity and anxiety
   B. a typical negative response to strangers
   C. her attempt to get warm in a damp environment
   D. A and B   (13:464)

187. Mary Lou is placed in a cool mist croupette. Which of the following would not apply in your nursing care?
   A. maintain a mist flow
   B. prevent chilling
   C. observe for signs of respiratory distress
   D. keep tubing filled with H_2O (13:461)

188. A tracheotomy is performed on Mary Lou to aid in the draining of secretions. Which of the following conditions may have indicated the procedure?
   A. prostration with severe cyanosis
   B. intense coughing
   C. restlessness
   D. hyperpyrexia   (13:460)

189. When caring for Mary Lou, what should be your primary concern?
   A. making friends with her
   B. controlling environment
   C. maintaining patent airway
   D. preventing accidents   (13:461)

190. Which of the following signs would indicate that Mary Lou's condition is guarded?
   A. restlessness, crying for mother, throwing away toys
   B. dyspnea, cyanosis, retractions, noisy respirations
   C. restlessness, fever, rapid pulse, pallor or cyanosis
   D. B and C   (13:460)

191. Which of the following equipment should be kept at Mary Lou's bedside?
   A. stethoscope, flashlight, blood pressure apparatus
   B. suction machine, emergency tray
   C. dextrose solution, I.V. stand
   D. B and C   (13:461)

192. In the care of the tracheostomy tube and incision you should
   A. use sterile gloves
   B. instill a few drops of sterile water into inner canula before removing it
   C. aspirate outer canula only
   D. A and C   (13:461)

193. If you are unable to aspirate the tracheobronchial tree successfully and respiratory difficulties persist, you should *immediately*
   A. instill a few drops of sterile saline solutions into canula
   B. remove inner canula if one is present
   C. take vital signs
   D. notify physician   (13:462)

194. If by accident the outer canula is removed from the trachea, which of the following should you do *first*?
   A. hold tracheotomy open with hemostat
   B. cleanse area with hydrogen peroxide
   C. summon physician
   D. A and C   (13:463)

195. Of the following toys, which would be most appropriate for Mary Lou to play with in her crib?
   A. picture book
   B. stuffed toy
   C. building blocks
   D. bubble pipe   (13:462)

196. In preparing the parents for Mary Lou's discharge, which of the following points should you emphasize in your health instructions?
   A. teach mother care of tracheostomy tube on Mary Lou
   B. teach mother care of tracheostomy tube on model
   C. caution mother concerning her child's playing in sandbox
   D. A and C   (13:464)

Alma Brown, 6 lbs. 4 oz., was born 2 hours ago and was noted to be in distress shortly after birth. The doctor attempted to pass a catheter from the nose to the stomach but was unable to do so. An x-ray taken immediately confirmed the diagnosis of a tracheoesophageal fistula; the type in which there is a blind upper pouch and a fistula from the lower segment of the esophagus to the trachea.

Answer items 197 through 202 based on the information given.

197. Other signs of a tracheoesophageal fistula which you would expect Alma to show are
    A. drooling, cyanosis, immediate regurgitation of feedings
    B. excessive crying, visible peristaltic waves, vomiting
    C. absence of meconium stool, vomiting, cyanosis
    D. weak cry, distention, projectile vomiting (13:204)

198. It is decided to operate on Alma immediately. Until Alma goes to the operating room you should
    1. suction her whenever necessary
    2. keep her in an isolette with oxygen and humidity
    3. keep her in Trendelenberg position to prevent aspiration
    4. give her glucose water until the anesthesiologist orders no further oral intake
    A. 1 and 2
    B. 1 and 4
    C. 2 and 3
    D. 3 and 4 (13:205)

199. Alma had a gastrostomy done immediately after the fistula was repaired. Later, in giving her gastrostomy feedings, the nurse should remember to
    1. give the infant a pacifier while she is receiving the feeding
    2. hold the syringe high above the baby's head to ensure enough pressure
    3. follow the formula with an equal amount of water
    4. place the infant on her side after the feeding
    5. keep the gastrostomy tube open but elevated when the feeding is finished
    A. 1, 2, and 3
    B. 1, 4, and 5
    C. 2, 3, and 4
    D. 3, 4, and 5 (13:205)

200. Alma continues to have moderate amounts of mucus in her nasopharynx and needs to be suctioned frequently. In postoperative suctioning you would
    1. use a #18 French catheter
    2. pass catheter back and forth rapidly several times to aspirate mucus
    3. insert catheter, aspirate mucus, and withdraw
    4. be certain no suction is applied while catheter is being inserted into the nasopharynx
    A. 1 and 2
    B. 1 and 3
    C. 2 and 4
    D. 3 and 4 (13:461)

201. The care of Alma's skin around the gastrostomy is exceedingly important. This area should be kept clean and
    A. covered with wet dressing
    B. covered with dry dressing
    C. protected with aluminum paste
    D. left uncovered (13:205)

202. If Alma had a cervical esophagostomy, which of the following measures is of fundamental importance?
    A. monthly check-ups
    B. referral to home nursing service
    C. "sham" feedings
    D. sucking a pacifier (13:205)

J. Skin Conditions

ACNE

Directions: This part of the test consists of a situation followed by a series of statements or questions. Study the situation and select the best answer to each statement or question that follows.

John Deer, a 16-year-old, has been seen in the clinic. His face and hair appear oily and there are numerous blackheads on the forehead and cheeks with some pitting. He is being seen in the clinic with the chief complaint of being "extremely tired" all of the time. He tells you, "A week ago I had a slight sore throat and a mild fever." Since then he has been sleeping as much as possible, but is always tired. "I can't keep up with my school work, basketball practice, church work and dates with my steady girl." The physical examination shows a temperature of 100.6° F, enlarged lymph nodes, spleen and liver. The doctor orders blood studies and bedrest for several days until reports are in.

Answer items 203 through 207 based on the information given.

203. From the history and physical findings, the possible diagnosis(es) is (are)
  A. tuberculosis
  B. infectious mononucleosis
  C. acne
  D. B and C   (13:701,717)

204. It is important to help John with this problem because you know that adolescents are
  A. more susceptible to secondary infection than younger children
  B. very diet conscious and you can take advantage of this for health teaching
  C. very sensitive about their appearances and how others see them
  D. A and B   (13:686)

205. Since John probably has an infectious condition, it is possible that he has exposed many people to his organisms. Which of the following contacts would be *most* susceptible?
  A. the basketball team
  B. his steady girl
  C. his family
  D. the church group   (13:686)

206. John is concerned about the skin condition of oiliness and blackheads. He asks you what causes this condition. You respond that there are many factors. Included in these might be
  A. familiar predisposition
  B. lack of sleep
  C. overactivity
  D. all of the above   (13:702)

207. He says, "But I didn't have trouble like this two years ago. It seems to have developed recently. Why?" Your *best* reply would be that
  A. nobody knows the reason why, but many adolescents have this kind of trouble for periods of time
  B. your body has changed and the increased secretions of male hormones increase oil gland activity
  C. this condition has undoubtedly been compounded by your mild upper respiratory condition
  D. the physiological changes during puberty cause this condition in all adolescents   (13:702)

ECZEMA

Directions: For each of the following **multiple choice questions, select the ONE most appropriate answer.**

208. Seven-month-old Jimmy is admitted to the hospital with eczema. His mother is quite concerned and asks you about the usual course of this illness. You know that most children
  A. have eczema until they reach the adolescent age
  B. outgrow it at around 4 years of age
  C. outgrow it but may show other allergic manifestations later in life
  D. have only one episode and then the condition disappears   (13:398)

209. Types of feedings which would be given to a child with eczema include
  1. an evaporated milk formula
  2. a soybean formula
  3. whole milk
  4. goat's milk
  A. 1 and 3
  B. 1 and 4
  C. 2 and 3
  D. 2 and 4   (13:401)

210. In planning Jimmy's nursing care, it is important that you
    1. use restraints to prevent his scratching
    2. give him frequent soap and water baths to increase his comfort
    3. use tender loving care and diversion to comfort him
    4. give him his favorite stuffed toy
    A. 4 and 2
    B. 4 and 3
    C. 2 and 1
    D. 3 and 1 (13:399)

211. To promote the maximum use of Jimmy's restraint, you should see to it that the restraint is
    A. removed every few hours
    B. applied snugly
    C. applied continuously
    D. applied on one arm at a time (13:399)

212. Infantile eczema is otherwise called
    A. scabies contagiosa
    B. atopic dermatitis
    C. skin allergy
    D. seborrhea (13:398)

213. Which of the following statements is *not* true of eczema?
    A. it is most frequent in the first two years of life
    B. it is uncommon in breast-fed infants
    C. it occurs frequently in female babies
    D. it is most frequent in well-nourished infants (13:398)

214. Which of the nursing measures below would best prevent irritation of the eczematous skin caused by rubbing against the sheet?
    A. use heavy plastic sheeting over cotton sheet
    B. bathe child in cornstarch water
    C. give oil bath before bedtime
    D. A and C (13:399)

215. What kind of diet would be best for an infant with eczema?
    A. bland diet
    B. ketogenic diet
    C. elimination diet
    D. regular diet (13:401)

216. In general, which of the following would be most appropriate for eczematous infants to play with?
    A. safe, soft, washable toys
    B. stuffed toys
    C. blocks, puzzles
    D. cloth remnants, paper dolls (13:401)

K. Other Situational Disorders

Directions: For each of the following multiple choice questions, select the ONE most appropriate answer.

217. Common signs of a brain tumor in a child are
    A. headache, diplopia
    B. convulsions, tachycardia
    C. ataxia, tachypnea
    D. nystagmus, decreased blood pressure (13:661)

218. In caring for a child in the immediate postoperative period following craniotomy, the nurse should
    A. allow her to assume the position most comfortable for her
    B. elevate her head 45° and keep her on the unoperative side
    C. keep her in Trendelenberg position on the operative side
    D. keep her flat on the unoperative side (13:663)

219. A child's postoperative period will be extremely difficult and trying for the parents. The nurse can help them to have a positive outlet for their feelings by
    1. obtaining the services of the hospital chaplain for them
    2. permitting them to assist in child care
    3. encouraging them to discuss their anxieties
    4. suggesting they read while the nurse cares for the child
    A. 1 and 2
    B. 1 and 4
    C. 2 and 3
    D. 3 and 4 (13:664,665)

Situational Problems

220. Postoperatively, which of the following would be expected of a child with a craniotomy?
    1. edema of the eyes
    2. dry conjunctivae
    3. high fever
    4. abdominal distention
    A. 1, 2 and 3
    B. 1, 2 and 4
    C. 1, 3 and 4
    D. 2, 3 and 4   (13:664)

221. In the preoperative care of a child with a Wilms' tumor, which of the following is *most* significant?
    A. keeping the child flat in bed
    B. providing a nutritious diet
    C. providing an adequate fluid intake
    D. cautioning against palpating the abdomen   (13:260)

222. Which of the following symptoms is *least* associated with brain tumors?
    A. increased blood pressure
    B. abdominal pain
    C. vomiting without nausea
    D. muscle weakness or paralysis   (13:661,662)

223. Which of the following *could* result from administering cortisone?
    A. hypertension, an increase in appetite, skin rash
    B. weight gain, anuria
    C. headache, vomiting and convulsions
    D. alopecia, fever, edema   (13:581,582)

224. You are aware that adolescents sometimes develop scoliosis. The type is frequently called
    A. idiopathic
    B. hereditary
    C. postural
    D. physiologic   (13:718)

225. Scoliosis could be defined as an exaggerated
    A. dorsal curvature of the thoracic region
    B. lateral curvature of the spinal column
    C. ventral curvature of the lumbar region
    D. dorsal curvature of the pelvic region   (13:718)

226. In working with blind children, the nurse should
    A. speak more frequently
    B. repeat conversation
    C. give child extra attention
    D. speak before touching child   (13:505)

227. Which of the senses must be maximally developed in totally blind children?
    A. touch
    B. taste
    C. hearing
    D. A and C   (13:504)

228. During the stage of edema in a child with an acute exacerbation of nephrosis, the parent and nurse should
    A. keep him on strict bedrest and amuse him with toys and quiet games
    B. keep him active and encourage a normal routine
    C. anticipate his needs, thereby decreasing both mental and physical frustrations
    D. change his position frequently and permit activity as tolerated   (13:488)

229. Which of the following symptoms are more characteristic of acute glomerulonephritis than nephrosis in children?
    1. hematuria
    2. hypertension
    3. proteinuria
    4. azotemia
    A. 1 and 2
    B. 1 and 3
    C. 2 and 4
    D. 3 and 4   (13:552)

230. The most important aspect of treatment for glomerulonephritis is
    A. bedrest
    B. low protein diet
    C. corticosteroids
    D. diuretics   (13:553)

231. The accumulation of fluid in the peritoneal cavity is called
    A. peritonitis
    B. ascites
    C. hydrothorax
    D. pleurisy   (13:486)

232. A nephrotic crisis during the course of nephrosis is associated with which of the following?
    A. hypertension
    B. azotemia
    C. abdominal pain
    D. hematuria (13:487)

233. In ABO incompatibility, the agglutinin of the mother's blood may affect the red blood cells of the fetus by causing
    A. clumping
    B. hemolysis
    C. coagulation
    D. sickling (13:196)

234. If an exchange transfusion is necessary in ABO incompatibility, the blood type used to exchange the newborn is
    A. A
    B. B
    C. O
    D. AB (13:196)

235. Rhogam is not indicated for treatment of an Rh-negative mother if the
    1. infant is Rh-positive
    2. infant is Rh-negative
    3. mother is sensitive to antigen
    4. father is Rh-positive
        A. 1 and 4
        B. 2 and 3
        C. 1 and 3
        D. 2 and 4 (13:195)

236. A positive direct Coombs' Test suggests that
    A. the mother has not been sensitized
    B. blood bilirubin levels are high
    C. antibodies are attached to fetal red blood cells
    D. antigens have not yet crossed placental barrier (13:196)

237. Tuberculosis is caused by
    A. an acid-fast bacillus
    B. an acid-fast coccus
    C. a gram-negative bacillus
    D. a gram-negative coccus (13:713)

238. When widespread tuberculosis infection occurs, the individual is said to have
    A. primary tuberculosis
    B. secondary tuberculosis
    C. infiltrating tuberculosis
    D. miliary tuberculosis (13:714)

239. Which of the following clinical manifestations is not present in primary tuberculosis?
    A. weight loss, fatigue
    B. anorexia, malaise
    C. hemoptysis, fever
    D. irritability, insomnia (13:715)

240. The test(s) used in the diagnosis of tuberculosis is (are) the
    A. Mantoux test
    B. Dick test
    C. Schick test
    D. A and C (13:715)

241. A positive tuberculin reaction in a child is usually evidence that he has any one of the following except
    A. a past tuberculosis infection
    B. an active lesion at time of testing
    C. an allergy to protein
    D. none of the above (13:715)

242. The most effective drug in common use against tuberculosis is
    A. PAS
    B. INH
    C. streptomycin
    D. kanamycin (13:716)

243. Infectious hepatitis is highly contagious and transmitted by
    A. fecal contamination
    B. droplet infection
    C. kissing
    D. contaminated needles (28:427)

244. Which of the following symptoms characterizes the onset of infectious hepatitis?
    A. weight loss, irritability, diplopia
    B. abdominal discomfort, vomiting, anorexia

C. jaundice, malaise, vomiting
D. A and C (28:427)

245. Management of patients with infectious hepatitis includes
A. ad lib diet with fat as tolerated
B. confinement to home
C. no restriction of activity
D. all of the above (28:428)

246. Which of the following is not true about tetanus neonatorum? (anaerobic)
A. it cannot be transmitted through contact
B. its causative organism is aerobic, spore-forming, gram-positive bacillus
C. isolation of infant is not necessary
D. its incubation period is 5 days to several weeks (13:220)

247. The clinical manifestations indicative of tetanus neonatorum include the following, except
A. opisthotonos
B. risus sardonicus
C. tonic-neck reflex — three mos. of life
D. trismus (13:220)

248. In planning for the care of the child with tetanus, your primary consideration should be
A. reduction of tactile and auditory stimuli
B. administration of sedatives
C. administration of oxygen
D. feeding of child (13:221)

249. Your nursing care of the aforenoted child should be
A. widely spaced
B. reduced to the minimum
C. planned around medication or treatment time
D. B and C (13:221)

250. The best way to feed a child with tetanus should be by
A. dropper
B. parenteral fluids
C. small feedings
D. gavage (13:221)

251. The prognosis of tetanus is very poor. Death is usually due to
A. aspiration pneumonia
B. exhaustion
C. respiratory failure
D. all of the above (13:221)

Directions: Match the following numbered items with the most appropriate lettered items.

B 252. Roundworm infestation (13:468)
A 253. Umbilical infection (13:219)
D 254. Acute glomerulonephritis (27:478)
C 255. Ringworm of scalp (13:634)

A. Escherichia coli
B. Ascaris lumbricoides
C. Microsporum audouini
D. Beta-hemolytic streptococci

C 256. Hematuria, convulsions, stiff neck, coma (13:392)
C 257. Severe pain in abdomen and legs (13:392)
A 258. Craniotabes (13:368)
B 259. Raw surface and intensely itchy area between toes (13:635)
D 260. Periorbital ecchymosis, epistaxis, bleeding from mouth (13:211)
A 261. Crouching, frog-like position (13:368)

A. Rickets
B. Tinea pedis
C. Sickle-cell anemia
D. Skull fracture

Chapter V: Answers and Explanations

1. **A.**—England was the first country to recognize the impact of hospitalization upon the child as a result of the separation from his family.
2. **D.**—Medical precaution and isolation techniques have been enforced in the hospital as indicated. This practice has essentially not been influenced by the advent of vaccination against contagious diseases.
3. **D.**—Preparation should be relevant to the child's forthcoming experience.
4. **D.**—Parents' involvement in the care of their hospitalized child has been found to be mutually satisfactory to both parents and child.
5. **A.**—Unnecessary hospitalization can result from insurance programs that provide reimbursement for health care obtained in an in-patient setting only.
6. **D.**—Health protection is most effective when it considers the totality of the needs of individuals.
7. **C.**—Toilet training would be a traumatic experience to a child within the first year of life.
8. **B.**—Playing with checkers and marbles is quite a hazard in infancy.
9. **D.**—If the aforenoted considerations could only be implanted, hospitalization would be a most meaningful experience for the child.
10. **A.**—Since play is a very important part of children's daily living, provision for indoor and outdoor space is important.
11. **D.**—The three aforenoted ways reflect ingenious ideas.
12. **D.**—School-age children are oriented to peer group activities and as such, a "secret" room may not be most appropriate for them.
13. **C.**—Talking of damage and repair of toys are ways that can help children deal with castration and mutilation fantasies common to this age group (phallic phase).
14. **A.**—This is especially significant to a child in this age group to allay undue anxiety.
15. **D.**—Fear of bodily mutilation is pronounced in the preschool years. For children under six, playful repetition to clarify the operative area for children may be used; for older children, direct explanations may be helpful.
16. **C.**—Such activity allows the child to express his anxiety and fear which may not be expressed otherwise.
17. **C.**—By giving conscious thought to his hospitalization, the child is prevented from repressing and retaining unrealistic fantasies.
18. **D.**—For children requiring frequent hospitalization, such measures facilitate future adjustment.
19. **B.**—The interdisciplinary team approach could be most useful only if the input of the team members were well coordinated.
20. **A.**—Even at this young age, verbal or play approaches can be most effective in preparing a child for hospitalization.
21. **D.**—Through play, the child can express his anxiety and demonstate a good deal of his coping mechanisms.
22. **C.**—Preparing a mother to stay with her child in the hospital is as important as preparing the child for the hospital experience.

However, the mother should be given a choice of whether or not to stay with her child in the hospital.
23. **B.**—The mother, or whoever is the child's significant other, is the child's natural source of support and separation can have a strong impact upon the child's sense of security.
24. **D.**—The enforced passivity and dependence during illness is greatly in conflict with the adolescent's efforts to establish independence and a sense of identity.
25. **D.**—The task may overwhelm the mother with all kinds of technical language which she is most unlikely to understand.
26. **A.**—Preparation for hospitalization is a process which continues throughout hospitalization with the ultimate aim of enabling child to achieve new strength and assurance for coping with future stress.
27. **C.**—By virtue of the rapid changes in the child's developmental system, children's responses to illness are oftentimes unpredictable.
28. **A.**—Finger painting is too advanced and watching television programs would be too tiring for a 2-year-old boy.
29. **A.**—Playing telephone and playing with pots and pans would give the child a feeling of closeness to home; a pounding board would help him express his anger.
30. **C.**—Such activity can provide an excellent outlet for the child's angry feelings.
31. **C.**—Acquainting parents with the different personality types of ward workers is rather an unprofessional task on the part of the nurse.
32. **D.**—Nurses should be personally secure and not respond subjectively to parents' statements.
33. **D.**—Disregard for ward policies is not a common expression of parental anxiety.
34. **C.**—Identifying the cause of anxiety and then giving parents whatever help the nurse can to relieve them of distress is most helpful.
35. **A.**—If the parents did make a mistake causing their child's illness, the nurse should help them recognize that mistakes can happen.
36. **D.**—Parental anxiety can be magnified by all the numerous factors associated with illness.
37. **B.**—Involving the mother in the care of her child during hospitalization can alleviate a great deal of her anxiety.
38. **C.**—Sensory deprivation can be prevented if provisions are made for close contact of child with another human being and the environment is sufficiently enriched.
39. **A.**—The aforenoted competencies are truly basic requirements in nursing of children and families.
40. **D.**—The child must not be permitted to harm other children even though he may be permitted to do so at home.
41. **A.**—The nurse should never be critical of a mother's attitude however unreasonable it may appear.
42. **A.**—The mother should be allowed to take her child to the unit accompanied by the nurse.
43. **B.**—Blood pressure taking does not have to be ordered by the physician. The nurse should know when blood pressure needs to be taken.
44. **B.**—Normal body temperature is 38° C or 98.6° F.
45. **D.**—The child should be made to feel that he could cry and react to pain when necessary.
46. **C.**—Such an approach can easily make a parent feel more guilty than ever.
47. **C.**—Medical aseptic technique is observed for all patients on admission with or without physician's advice.
48. **A.**—Terminal disinfection is done upon discharge of the patient.
49. **C.**—Once a mask is wet it should be discarded whether or not it has just been worn. Moist medium favors growth of pathogens.
50. **C.**—The nurse in any shared nurse-parent learning situation at the hospital must consider the special needs of the parents. While they may be encouraged to participate in the care of their hospitalized child, they should never be required to do so if they are not feeling sufficiently comfortable to assume the responsibility.
51. **D.**—The 10-year-old child is entering the age when the need for group approval and

a sense of achievement are at their highest points.
52. **B.**—The adolescent is in the stage of accepting a new body image as well as getting emancipated from the parents. Anything that threatens her ability to accomplish these tasks will be anxiety-producing.
53. **C.**—1 cc = 15 min. Proceed to solve, using the formula:
$$\frac{\text{desired dose}}{\text{dose on hand}} \times \text{dilutant} = \text{amount to be given}$$
54. **B.**—The fear of death is the most inescapable of all the fears faced by the living.
55. **B.**—Nurse should try to maintain the infant's sense of security.
56. **D.**—Illness and/or hospitalization represents a crisis to which families may have varied responses.
57. **C.**—If the mother has not prepared the child before he comes to the hospital, she is probably incapable of doing so. The nurse must then explain to the child in understandable language what will be done in the operating room and how he will feel when he comes out of anesthesia.
58. **C.**—These are symptoms indicative of hemorrhage.
59. **D.**—Play is a good catharsis.
60. **A.**—Hospitalization could be a very threatening situation to some children; under this condition a child may resort to earlier modes of behavior or cling to familiar objects for a sense of security.
61. **D.**—Upon being hospitalized, the toddler experiences basic fears: loss of love, fear of the unknown and fear of punishment. This sequence of responses to anaclitic depression has been cited in studies by Spitz and Bowlby.
62. **D.**—The child appears to be displaying a behavior reflective of despair.
63. **A.**—Medical rounds with discussions at the bedside ignores the individuality of the patient.
64. **B.**—Understanding the procedure would lessen the child's fear of the unknown.
65. **A.**—Respirations are difficult and irregular. They may be rapid and shallow.
66. **B.**—Vigorous measures may cause the infant to gasp once or twice, but are not helpful in establishing respiration.
67. **C.**—A perceptive, understanding nurse can do a great deal in allaying the parents' fear and anxiety concerning the care of their premature baby.
68. **B.**—The blood vessels of the premature infant are incompletely developed and therefore more fragile; the supporting tissue lacks normal elasticity and the plasma is hypothrombinemic.
69. **B.**—High arterial oxygen tension is a potent contributory factor probably through its effect on the developing vasculature.
70. **C.**—Ideally, the infant's body temperature should be 98°F but stability of temperature is more important than maintaining it at exactly 98°F.
71. **D.**—Nutritional problems in the premature infant are complicated by his difficulty in sucking and swallowing.
72. **B.**—Prematures, for a variety of reasons (lack of fatty tissue, immature temperature-regulatory center in the brain, immature circulation) cannot adequately regulate their own temperature.
73. **A.**—This condition is due to dilation of the blood vessels of the retina; after the vessels become excessively tortuous the retina may become detached, causing blindness. A relationship has been seen between the preceding condition and increased partial pressure of O_2 in the retinal arteries due to an O_2-rich atmosphere of over 40%.
74. **C.**—Contaminated hands are a prime method of transmitting infection between infants.
75. **C.**—Glucuronyl transferase is required to produce water soluble bilirubin, which can be excreted via the kidneys. Therefore, when this activity is diminished the unconjugated bilirubin is deposited in the skin and mucous membranes.
76. **B.**—Because the infant is receiving no visual stimuli and has limited tactile stimuli as a result of lying nude in his bed, the nurse must supply this stimulation.
77. **C.**—These are best metabolized by the newborn for energy.
78. **A.**—Extensive studies have been accom-

plished to study the mother-child relationship and the effects of separation on the establishment of this relationship.
79. **B.**—Intubation through the nose obstructs adequate exchange of gases.
80. **B.**—The premature requires a minimum of 120–130 cal/kg. per day and 130–150 ml./kg. of water for adequate hydration and nutrition to meet their special needs. The normal newborn requires a minimum of 110–130 cal./kg. per day from his formula and 75–90 ml./kg. of water.
81. **A.**—These infants are from 20 to 27 weeks gestation and are generally incapable of extrauterine existence.
82. **C.**—The child of a diabetic may be born prematurely due to excessive weight gain by infant due to placental transfer of glucose from mother in utero and inability of the mother's uterus to carry the large infant. A mother with incompetency of the cervix is unable to carry the fetus to term due to injury or congenital weakness of the cervical os.
83. **B.**—The infant has thin and delicate mucous membranes, rendering him susceptible to infection, injury, and insensible water loss. He produces decreased amounts of surfactant and his liver activity is immature. The disproportionate loss of fluid in an infant increases the hazards of electrolyte imbalance. Capillary fragility predisposes the infant to injury and cerebral hemorrhage.
84. **A.**—The spastic diplegic or quadriplegic cerebral palsy is a common abnormal finding among premature babies.
85. **C.**—The nurse should recognize the complexity of the problem and start with the family's own resources when working out solutions.
86. **A.**—It is extremely important that parents perceive the child's problems realistically and receive guidance in handling them effectively.
87. **D.**—Never keep a premature baby lying flat on his back while feeding for there is a great danger of aspirating the spit-up substances.
88. **A.**—The mouth, which is the pleasure zone in the first year of life, is also used by the infant as a means of aggression.
89. **C.**—Hyperventilation may result in respiratory alkalosis which leads to confusion and coma.
90. **B.**—A metabolic acidosis is also found due to renal compensation leading to loss of base from the body.
91. **D.**—All the aforenoted measures are attempts to eliminate the salicylates from Jimmy's system. Gavage will wash out any salicylate contents from the stomach; the syrup of ipecac will stimulate the child to vomit and parenteral fluids will speed the excretion of salicylates in the urine.
92. **D.**—The toddler is entering the age of developing autonomy and, as such, has great curiosities about the world around him.
93. **C.**—Social development occurs when the toddler participates in activity with other children.
94. **D.**—Scotch tape test is usually done early in the morning for the purpose of locating the eggs of the pinworm. Anal swabbing is best done in the early morning before arising or just before dressing, bathing, or defecating.
95. **B.**—Oxyuriasis is spread by person-to-person contact.
96. **C.**—Vaginitis often occurs, and insomnia, too.
97. **C.**—That is irrelevant in home situations. The measure is applicable to the hospital setting.
98. **D.**—Parent education is an effective means of preventing accidents at home.
99. **D.**—Those are corrosives and vomiting would only spread the substance to other parts of the stomach, throat and mouth.
100. **C.**—Communicable diseases which claimed the heaviest toll of young lives in the early twentieth century are now near the bottom of the list of causes of death.
101. **B.**—Accidents far outnumber all other causes of death among children and young adults.
102. **B.**—The death rate from drowning among boys is four times greater than that of girls.
103. **B.**—The preadolescent period appears to be the age at which biking is most popular

and where young adolescents are strongly competitive with each other and tend to be group oriented even at the sacrifice of personal safety.
104. **C.**—The area is red, blistered, and extremely painful.
105. **B.**—A second-degree burn may result in eschar formation.
106. **A.**—Contracting scars must not be allowed to form during the healing stage.
107. **C.**—Abdominal discomfort or bleeding of the gastrointestinal tract indicates a stress or Curling's ulcer, which may occur in burned patients.
108. **C.**—The sympathetic and insightful nurse can do a lot to relieve the child of his distress. She should allow the child to express his feelings.
109. **D.**—The nurse should recognize the importance of allowing the child to express his hostility and anger; the use of a puppet is appealing to toddlers.
110. **B.**—Intrusive procedures involving the perineal area may cause considerable distress to preschoolers.
111. **C.**—Preschool children are fearful of bodily harm during hospitalization and since they have only a limited knowledge of body functions, they fantasize about what is happening "inside."
112. **D.**—Preschoolers would not be too happy playing with school-age boys because of marked developmental differences.
113. **C.**—The five-year-old child knows enough about the passage of time to realize that if he waits, his mother will come back at some fairly definite time.
114. **D.**—The nurse should respect the individuality of children.
115. **A.**—The preschool child's level of understanding has an important bearing on his responses to illness and hospitalization. They are generally fearful of bodily harm.
116. **B.**—Preschoolers have many fantasies about bodily functions since they have only a limited knowledge. Fear of mutilation is common in this age group.
117. **D.**—The cited measures are extremely important, especially if the child has a long period of hospitalization.
118. **A.**—The aforenoted first aid treatment is helpful in controlling pain, fluid loss, and infections.
119. **D.**—Renal blood flow is lessened just when it is needed to clear potassium and nitrogenous components of the dead cells in the burned area.
120. **D.**—In the treatment of second and third-degree burns, the first step is to combat shock.
121. **A.**—Susy's diet should also be high in vitamins, particularly vitamin C and iron for tissue repair.
122. **B.**—Parents may feel guilty because of lack of supervision of the child, which would have prevented his injury. Both the child and his parents need reassurance and understanding.
123. **B.**—Ten-year-old children enjoy engaging in activities that are creative.
124. **C.**—Hero worship is intense at this age.
125. **D.**—Ten-year-olds desire perfection in their complex abilities and competition is fairly strong.
126. **C.**—To preadolescent children, negative requests afront their sense of personal worth.
127. **A.**—Failure to develop a sense of industry will lead the child to acquire or intensify earlier feelings of inferiority and inadequacy.
128. **D.**—Fracture of the femur will not affect the symmetry of the shoulders.
129. **C.**—Most simple fractures are treated by closed manipulation traction or casting.
130. **B.**—The fundamental principle of this traction system is a bilateral Buck's extension applied to the legs.
131. **C.**—After traction has been applied to the child's legs, it should be checked carefully in order to prevent constriction of circulation or injury to the feet. Warm dry toes would indicate free circulation in and to the feet.
132. **B.**—Episodic abdominal pain may occur owing to the enlarged lymph node.
133. **D.**—Supportive measures to promote comfort in the care of a leukemic child cannot be overemphasized.
134. **D.**—The platelet count in leukemic children is very much lowered and is largely

responsible for hemorrhagic manifestations.
135. **B.**—The production of normal blood cells is rapidly reduced hence the platelet count is low.
136. **A.**—The child should be told the purpose and details of the procedure.
137. **C.**—The child should not be treated too permissively or be overindulged just because she is ill.
138. **B.**—The nurse must gain the trust of both the child and her parents so that she can help them through these traumatic experiences.
139. **D.**—Vincristine may cause constipation, footdrop, and alopecia.
140. **D.**—Anxiety may predispose another bout of bleeding.
141. **B.**—The child tires easily and therefore needs frequent rest periods.
142. **B.**—Hemarthrosis and hemorrhage into the joints are the hallmarks of hemophilia.
143. **C.**—The nurse must remain with the parents at the dying child's bedside to assure them that everything possible is being done for the child's comfort.
144. **C.**—In leukemia, it may be more than 50,000 per cubic millimeter.
145. **A.**—Otherwise, death results from the disease itself or from concurrent infections or both.
146. **C.**—No cure is known and treatment is altogether palliative, supportive, and specific.
147. **C.**—In the acute phase of rheumatic fever, rest is all important to reduce the work of the heart.
148. **C.**—The level of the antibody response reflects the intensity of tissue reaction. The common focus of infection is in the throat or skin.
149. **B.**—The three principal clinical manifestations of rheumatic fever are carditis, migratory polyarthritis and Sydenham's chorea.
150. **D.**—Sore joints should be handled carefully when child is moved.
151. **D.**—The child may have anorexia, vomiting, sweating, and hyperpyrexia.
152. **A.**—Sydenham's chorea is the other major manifestation of rheumatic fever.
153. **D.**—The important thing is to immediately put the child under a regimen of treatment once he has been observed demonstrating signs and symptoms of the disease.
154. **D.**—Recreational therapy should be geared to the child's developmental level and interests.
155. **C.**—Recurrence must be prevented since each attack increases the threat of additional cardiac damage.
156. **A.**—The child's activities must be confined to the limits permitted by the physician.
157. **B.**—The child should be kept from persons with upper respiratory infections. The prevention of recurrences of rheumatic fever lies in the prevention of infection with group A beta hemolytic streptococci.
158. **C.**—An insightful nurse is very reassuring. Parents should be helped in finding solutions to many of the management problems as they occur. Oftentimes, anticipatory counseling is quite helpful.
159. **B.**—Sydenham's chorea is most common in girls from 7 to 14 years of age.
160. **B.**—Both treatment and nursing care are based on the relief of symptoms. The child should have absolute physical and mental rest.
161. **D.**—Its onset is gradual; the first sign may be clumsiness.
162. **D.**—Cardiac failure rarely occurs after the age of six months.
163. **B.**—Referral could be done by convenient appointment.
164. **C.**—Observations to note are whether the cyanosis is circumoral or equally distributed over the body, and the like.
165. **D.**—The technique is performed using the stethoscope.
166. **B.**—The infant is cyanotic instead.
167. **B.**—If the ductus is large and much blood is shunted into the pulmonary circulation, there may be retardation in growth.
168. **A.**—If the pulse and respiratory rates rise and the blood pressure drops, and if the child is very thirsty, the child is likely to be hemorrhaging.
169. **A.**—The arterial blood is not normally saturated with oxygen thus giving a bluish tint to the skin. Squatting relieves the strain of standing.

170. **B.**—Many cardiologists prefer the increased flexibility of digoxin when digitalis is no longer required in the presence of toxicity.
171. **B.**—The drug is completely absorbed in the gastrointestinal tract so there are no potential difficulties in dosage.
172. **B.**—Careful observation of the vital signs of children on digitalis therapy cannot be overemphasized.
173. **D.**—There are four associated anomalies in tetralogy of Fallot, namely, a valvular pulmonary stenosis, interventricular septal defect, dextroposition of aorta, and hypertrophy of the right ventricle.
174. **D.**—This procedure is done under either general or local anesthesia.
175. **D.**—Any indication of irregularities in the vital signs must be reported at once to the physician.
176. **D.**—These three types of congenital heart diseases are acyanotic; however, if the anomaly is such that venous blood eventually mixes with arterial blood when the heart weakens, cyanosis may result.
177. **A.**—The symptoms of patent ductus arteriosus in infants are usually so slight that the condition is not discovered at the initial sign.
178. **C.**—Chest drainage must be observed accurately for color, amount, and consistency.
179. **B.**—Coughing should be encouraged to prevent retention of secretion and atlectasis and to promote lung expansion.
180. **D.**—The bedside nurse should be alert to observe signs of pneumothorax which are restlessness, apprehension, cyanosis, sudden sharp chest pain, tachycardia and dyspnea.
181. **A.**—The child is ready to assume more responsibility for his own care and to play with other children. The parents must be helped to find other satisfactions to replace those of caring for an ill child.
182. **A.**—The nurse should recognize that infants, like adults may suffer congestive heart failure suddenly or it may be predictable.
183. **A.**—The air blockage can then result in overdistention of the lung, dyspnea and cyanosis.
184. **B.**—The onset may be sudden and accompanied by prostration, hyperpyrexia and severe dyspnea.
185. **B.**—The potential traumatic effects of hospitalization upon the child can be greatly minimized by allowing her to hold on to familiar objects and persons.
186. **A.**—In this situation, the nurse can encourage the child to express her feelings and provide support for her.
187. **D.**—Control of the environment is important in the prevention of emergency situations.
188. **A.**—Other indications for tracheotomy are signs of cardiac failure and restricted expansion of the lungs.
189. **C.**—Maintenance of the artificial airway is of fundamental importance, all the rest follows.
190. **D.**—When those signs are observed, the nurse must immediately check the condition of the tracheostomy, and at the same time call for the doctor.
191. **B.**—A sterile tray should also be kept at the bedside for routine care of the tracheostomy tube.
192. **A.**—The nurse should aspirate the outer canula and tracheobronchial tree, although the depth to which she is permitted to aspirate the tracheobronchial tree depends on the medical policy.
193. **D.**—The physician should be notified immediately, so that the lower airway can be investigated.
194. **A.**—The tracheotomy must be kept open with a hemostat while another nurse summons a doctor.
195. **B.**—A stuffed toy such as a teddy bear or a cat can encourage the child to express her feelings. Therefore, after her own hospital procedure she may express her feelings through her toy.
196. **D.**—The child may be discharged before the tracheostomy tube has been removed, thus the mother must be gradually taught by demonstration the care of the child before she leaves the hospital. Playing in the sandbox should be discouraged because of the danger of aspiration.
197. **A.**—Delivery nurses should be alerted to a newborn who readily gets cyanotic following suction of secretions from nose and

Situational Problems

mouth. The presence of excess mucus should be reported at once.

198. **A.**—The infant needs the individual attention of a nurse because frequent suctioning is necessary.
199. **B.**—Sucking on the nipple is quite significant for the child since it provides her with normal sucking pleasure, exercise for her jaw muscles, and relaxation while being fed.
200. **D.**—The aspiratory catheter should be pinched so that the lumen is closed while it is inserted into the opening of the outer tube.
201. **C.**—Displacement of tube when dressing must be prevented.
202. **C.**—"Sham" feeding of strained food after 2 months of age, so that the child can become used to various tastes and textures as she grows, even though she cannot digest the food.
203. **D.**—The two cited conditions are among the common health problems of adolescents.
204. **C.**—Feeling weak and less capable physically and physiologically will be quite threatening to the adolescent's pride and self-concept.
205. **B.**—Infectious mononucleosis is otherwise known as the "kissing disease."
206. **D.**—It is rather difficult to pinpoint any one specific cause of acne. Acne should be treated as early as possible since this skin condition can produce scars.
207. **B.**—The glands then become dilated, the pores become darkened from dirt accumulation, and bacteria thrive in the retained material.
208. **C.**—Eczema is the most frequent evidence of allergy seen in infancy.
209. **D.**—Vitamins C and D must be added with any substitute formula.
210. **D.**—Restraints are important in local treatment, but should be applied only when necessary. Stuffed toys should be discouraged as they could be a source of allergens.
211. **A.**—The restraint should be removed every few hours to allow free movement.
212. **B.**—Seborrhea and diaper rash may be frequently associated with infantile eczema.
213. **C.**—Eczema occurs in both sexes, in any race, and at any season.
214. **A.**—In this way, the baby can be turned from side to side and lie upon his back without putting undue pressure on the lesions.
215. **C.**—If the infant is on an elimination diet, he should be given a list of foods he may have rather than a list of foods to be avoided.
216. **A.**—The toys must have a smooth surface. Stuffed toys which contain wool, feathers, or kapok should not be used.
217. **A.**—Most of the symptoms are due to increased intracranial pressure.
218. **D.**—After the danger of vomiting has passed his position should be changed frequently from side to side to prevent pressure sores and hypostatic pneumonia.
219. **C.**—Parents could be greatly helped by a nurse who is insightful, knowledgeable, and competent.
220. **A.**—Hyperthermia may be caused by intracranial edema, bleeding or disturbance of the heat regulating center.
221. **D.**—Manipulating the abdominal wall inadvertently increases the danger of metastasis.
222. **B.**—Changes in vital signs are important in diagnosing increased intracranial pressure.
223. **D.**—Alopecia could be most disturbing to adolescents and older children.
224. **A.**—Scoliosis is usually found in young girls.
225. **B.**—Scoliosis is most frequent between the ages of 12 and 16 years, a period of rapid growth.
226. **D.**—Blind children can interpret people's moods by the inflection of their voice.
227. **D.**—The senses of touch and hearing of the blind child can be exploited to compensate for his lack of sight.
228. **A.**—Complete bed rest is necessary only during severe edema and when other symptoms are present.
229. **A.**—The urine may be grossly bloody or may have a smoky color.
230. **A.**—The treatment is symptomatic. During the acute phase, bed rest is all important.

231. **B.**—Ascites and hydrothorax are common symptoms of nephrosis.
232. **C.**—At times, the crisis is associated with erysipeloid skin eruptions.
233. **A.**—The difficulty is caused by the presence of the blood group A and B factors.
234. **C.**—Exchange transfusion is done if the infant's serum bilirubin reaches more than 20 mg. per 100 ml.
235. **C.**—Another point against the use of Rhogam is that it is expensive.
236. **C.**—In this situation, the mother's blood is Rh-negative and the infant's Rh-positive.
237. **A.**—The organism is called Mycobacterium tuberculosis.
238. **D.**—This type generally occurs in the infant or very young child.
239. **C.**—Hemoptysis and fever appear in the secondary stage of tuberculosis.
240. **A.**—Two other tests used for the same purpose are the tine test and the Heaf multiple puncture test.
241. **D.**—The test does not necessarily mean that the person has an active tuberculous process. A positive diagnosis of tuberculosis is made if the tubercle bacillus is found in the gastric contents or sputum.
242. **B.**—INH has a low toxicity and is effective in preventing hematogenous dissemination.
243. **A.**—It occurs most commonly in young adults.
244. **B.**—Jaundice appears several days later.
245. **D.**—There is no specific therapy.
246. **B.**—Its causative organism is *anaerobic* and as such develops only when it is not exposed to the air.
247. **C.**—Tonic-neck reflex is an expected behavior during the first three months of life.
248. **A.**—Unnecessary handling and noise should be avoided to prevent convulsion.
249. **C.**—This is primarily to minimize tactile and auditory stimulation.
250. **D.**—Since the child is heavily sedated it is necessary to feed him by gavage.
251. **D.**—The mortality rate is up to 50% of the cases.
252. **B.**—The worms are found most commonly in the lumen of the small intestines.
253. **A.**—Umbilical infection can also be caused by other pyogenic organisms.
254. **D.**—Acute glomerulonephritis may be due to hypersensitivity to an extrarenal infection with certain types of the aforenoted pathogens.
255. **C.**—The infection is highly contagious.
256. **C.**—The disease is confined almost exclusively to Negroes.
257. **C.**—Jaundice may appear two to three days after the crisis.
258. **A.**—An outstanding sign of advanced rickets becomes primarily apparent in the occipital bones.
259. **B.**—Pain may follow if child rubs or scratches the area.
260. **D.**—The diagnosis of skull fracture is made on the basis of roentgenograms of the skull.
261. **A.**—Bowlegs or knock-knees, accompanied by flat feet, are probably the most obvious deformities.

CHAPTER VI

Social Problems

INTRODUCTION

Growing concerns in the child health care field include the increasing prevalence of child abuse, drug abuse, venereal diseases, and juvenile delinquency; problems which cut across cultural barriers. There is indeed an urgent need to know how parents, children, health workers, and society as a whole, share the responsibility for the many social problems confronting mankind today and how people can work together to resolve these problems.

Nursing plays a very important role in the preventive and restorative aspects of society's health status. To enable the nurse to play her role effectively, it is necessary that she possess substantial knowledge concerning the nature of societal problems, their corresponding physiological and psychosocial dynamics, and the basic principles underlying nursing intervention. It is thus anticipated that the review questions contained in this chapter will enhance your understanding of prevailing social problems and, consequently, help you to gain further insight into these problems. This chapter aims to help you facilitate health care and intervene in crisis situations.

A. Child Abuse

Directions: This part of the test consists of a situation followed by a series of statements or questions. Study the situation and select the best answer to each statement or question that follows.

Jenny, a two and one-half-year-old child, is seen in the emergency room. She has a black eye and hematoma on the right forehead and her right arm hangs limply at her side. She appears to be small, her height is 29 inches and she weighs 20 pounds. She cries hard when the nurse approaches her, and she screams and kicks when the doctor examines her. Jenny is just beginning to walk by herself. Her mother says she usually plays in a playpen and sleeps "a lot." She will feed herself cookies, but will not use a spoon to feed herself. Her appetite is "poor." When asked how Jenny hurt herself, her mother says, "She fell out of her highchair. The babysitter turned her back and she fell."

Answer items 1–10 based on the information given.

1. From the history, you might consider that Jenny may be suffering from
   A. battered child syndrome
   B. failure to thrive syndrome
   C. maternal deprivation
   D. all of the above   (19:408,409)

2. Jenny is admitted. You are assigned to her care. In planning this care you will
   A. place her with older children for meals to learn to feed herself
   B. arrange for no visiting since she is upset by her mother

     (C.) request to be assigned to her on a continuous basis
     D. teach proper childrearing practices to mother   (13:409)

3. You are selecting a toy for Jenny. Which toy would be most appropriate for her?
   A. push toy
   B. blocks
   (C.) picture books
   D. pot and lid   (13:438)

4. Jenny is found to have a severe iron deficiency anemia. The *most* important nursing concern in this case is to
   A. help the child to ambulate
   B. teach proper diet to mother
   (C.) conserve the child's energy
   D. observe for respiratory distress   (13:389,390)

5. The most guarded complication of anemia a nurse should watch for is
   A. jaundice
   B. urinary retention
   C. respiratory infection
   (D.) congestive heart failure   (19:244)

6. You are developing a nursing care plan for Jenny. Your primary concern should be directed toward
   A. provision of emotionally supportive care
   B. establishing positive relation between mother and child
   C. care of her injuries
   (D.) A and C   (19:409)

7. Your long-term goals for Jenny should include the following, *except*
   A. teaching her what and how to eat
   (B.) alerting police department concerning child's family situation
   C. developing her gross and fine motor coordination
   D. encouraging her to play with own age group   (19:409)

8. Your charting from the time of Jenny's admission should include the following, *except*
   A. observations of child's condition
   B. doctor's orders which have been carried out
   C. mother's statements about her having beaten Jenny
   (D.) your judgment that child had been beaten   (19:409)

9. In planning for Jenny's snacks which of the following foods should you eliminate?
   A. buttermilk
   B. orange juice
   (C.) soda
   D. ice cream   (7:65)

10. During Jenny's subsequent stay in the hospital, which of the following activities would be the *least* beneficial to her?
   (A.) watching television programs alone
   B. regimented physical exercise
   C. playing with blocks in playroom
   D. "strolling" down hospital corridors with nurse   (13:418,419)

Directions: For each of the following multiple choice questions, select the ONE most appropriate answer.

11. Battering parents generally reveal the following characteristics, *except*
   (A.) liking to be alone
   B. feeling pressure about doing a good job
   C. being generally sensitive about their general ability and effectiveness as parents
   D. displaying no positive feelings about the child   (12:150)

12. There is general agreement that the basic essence of child abuse is
   A. superego identification with the parent's own punitive parent
   (B.) high parental demand combined with disregard of the infant's own needs, limited abilities, and helplessness
   C. a healthy desire to do something good for the infant
   D. a deep yearning for the child to respond in such a way as to bolster the parent's low self-esteem   (12:130)

Social Problems

13. A nurse working with an abusing parent should basically
    A. not accept parent's initial attitudes to her at face value
    B. focus her attention almost exclusively on the parent
    C. listen sympathetically to what the parent says
    D. resolve her own feelings about a parent who has hurt a small child (12:138)

14. A parent's aggressive acts toward children are generally a symptom of deep conflict and can best be controlled by
    A. separating the child from the abusing parent
    B. treating the symptoms
    C. change of environment
    D. dealing with parent's total personality (12:139)

15. "Role reversal" is defined as a reversal of the dependency role in which a parent may
    A. expect and demand a great deal from his (her) small children
    B. turn to his small children for nurturing and protection
    C. perceive the child as the psychotic portion of the parent which the parent wishes to control or destroy
    D. project much of his (her) difficulty onto the child (12:109)

16. The distribution pattern of child abuse incidents reported in accordance with the law is likely to be a biased reflection of actual distribution patterns. Which of the following may not be a reason for the distortion?
    A. variations in identifying and reporting child abuse incidents among different social subsegments of the population
    B. interstate differences of reporting laws
    C. intrastate variations of compliance with reporting provisions of the laws
    D. restricted variation of cases being reported on child abuse (12:22)

17. Which of the following is not true concerning the problem of child abuse?
    A. the methods used in infanticide have not changed much throughout history
    B. urbanization and the machine age have led to other forms of child abuse and to increasing mortality
    C. abuse of children has persistently excited increasing sympathy from the general public
    D. illegitimacy is a prime cause of infanticide (12:15)

18. Successful treatment of child abusers may be reflected in
    A. change in the style of parent-child interaction to a degree which eliminates the danger of physical and emotional harm
    B. improvement in marital and other interpersonal relationships
    C. improvement in dealing with various problems of daily living
    D. all of the above (12:138)

19. In order to most effectively resolve the problem of child abuse, it may be necessary to involve the
    A. psychiatrist, police department, social service agency
    B. pediatrician, nurses, church, roentgenologist
    C. family, public health department, school
    D. all of the above (12:143)

20. Which one of the following situations may not justify a law enforcement agency to take a battered child into protective custody?
    A. when only one parent has abused the child
    B. when both parents have only abused the child slightly
    C. when the nonparticipating parent does not sympathize with the violator
    D. when there are no responsible adults available to assume care and custody of the victim (12:3)

B. Drug Abuse

Directions: Match the following numbered items with the most appropriate lettered items.

21. A powerfully addictive opiate (6:48)
22. Produced from a hemp plant (6:34)

D 23. Masks the symptoms of fatigue (6:46)
C 24. Popularly known as "horse," "smack," "junk" (6:48)
B 25. Commonly known as "love drug" (6:43)
D 26. Chronic use leads to increasing tension, irritability, aggression (6:46)
C 27. Addiction starts with sniffing substance, proceeds to skin popping, then continues on to main-lining (6:49)
B 28. "Flashbacks" may recur spontaneously several days or months following its use (6:43)
A 29. Commonly known as "pot," "grass," "tea," "dope" (6:34)
B 30. Produces hallucinatory effects (6:42)
  A. Marijuana
  B. L.S.D.
  C. Heroin
  D. Amphetamines

Directions: For each of the following multiple choice questions, select the ONE most appropriate answer.

31. Which of the following is a documented statement about marijuana?
  (A.) marijuana does not produce physical dependency and is, therefore, nonaddictive
  B. marijuana usually leads to the use of more dangerous drugs
  C. many heroin addicts are known to have been heavy smokers of marijuana
  D. marijuana inevitably sets the user on a course towards addiction to hard drugs (6:39)

32. A widely known mind-altering drug is
  A. codeine
  B. phenobarbital
  (C.) mescaline
  D. benzedrine (6:42)

33. An example of a "down" drug is
  (A.) equanil
  B. benzedrine
  C. cocaine
  D. nicotine (6:47)

34. What drug is otherwise known as "speed" or "crystal"?
  A. benzedrine
  B. dexedrine
  (C.) methedrine
  D. equanil (6:46)

35. Which of the following drugs is usually dissolved in fruit drinks or added to food such as cookies and sugar cubes?
  (A.) L.S.D.
  B. benzedrine
  C. cocaine
  D. methedrine (6:41,42)

36. Which of the following measures is *least* effective in the prevention of drug addiction?
  A. encouraging drug education in the schools as early as possible
  B. discouraging advertisers from touting drugs as panaceas for all human problems
  C. educating parents to talk with, not at, their children
  (D.) encouraging parents to be pals with their children (6:38)

37. Sensory experiences of a person under L.S.D. may include the following sensations, *except*
  A. feeling that his body is dissolving
  B. feeling that he is going insane
  C. seeing colors explode, objects bend and flow
  (D.) an intense aversion to music (6:42)

Directions: The following items pertain to the effects of heroin upon the human organism. Match the following numbered items with the most appropriate letttered items.

B 38. Period of drowsiness (6:49)
D 39. Slowing down of mental and physical activities for two or three hours (6:49)
A 40. "Push" lasting only about a minute (6:49)
C 41. "On the nod" (6:49)
  A. Instantaneous sensation of pleasurable feeling
  B. Follows the initial response to heroin
  C. Appearing like someone who is fast asleep
  D. Sharp edges of reality are blurred

Directions: For each of the following multiple choice questions, select the ONE most appropriate answer.

42. A factor that is *not* a major reason cited by drug abusers for use of illicit drugs is
    A. pleasure
    B. curiosity
    C. peer group influence
    D. parental use of drugs   (18:12,13)

43. Which of the following risk factors has the *least* impact upon illicit drug use?
    A. low self-esteem
    B. mother or father uses marijuana
    C. drug use by many close friends
    D. favors legalization of marijuana (18:13)

44. Which of the following is *not* true about smoking and drug abuse?
    A. any regular use of cigarettes or alcohol, regardless of the amount, markedly increases likelihood of concurrent or subsequent use of an illicit drug
    B. many cured nonsmoking heroin addicts become very heavy cigarette smokers
    C. those who become involved in the drug scene are more likely to be practicing no religion
    D. parents, who are heavy smokers, markedly increase likelihood of children's illicit drug use   (18:14,15)

45. Which of the following is *not true* about drug abuse among adolescents?
    A. widespread heroin abuse is more a phenomenon of the urban ghetto
    B. hallucinogen abuse is more common in suburban and college communities
    C. inhalation of volatile hydrocarbons is limited almost exclusively to the younger adolescent
    D. female adolescent drug abusers appear to outnumber males by approximately three to one   (18:23)

46. Skin-popping of heroin frequently leads to the following consequences, *except*
    A. cellulitis
    B. occlusive thrombophlebitis
    C. abscess formation
    D. subcutaneous fat necrosis   (18:23)

47. Both marijuana and the amphetamines will cause
    A. tachycardia and hypertension within 30 minutes
    B. bradycardia and hypertension within 30 minutes
    C. cardiac arrhythmia
    D. pulmonary hypertension and right ventricular failure   (18:27)

48. The most significant somatic consequence of drug abuse affecting the heart is
    A. pericarditis
    B. myocarditis
    C. endocarditis
    D. myocardial infarction   (18:27)

49. Which of the following groups of signs and symptoms may accompany the use of hallucinogenic agents?
    A. nausea, vomiting, diarrhea, and abdominal pain
    B. headaches, anorexia, constipation, and abdominal pain
    C. double vision, vertigo, diarrhea, and vomiting
    D. constipation, abdominal pain, nausea, and vomiting   (18:30)

50. The following gynecologic conditions are commonly found among heroin addicted adolescent girls, *except*
    A. cervical erosion
    B. secondary amenorrhea
    C. vesicular or ulcerative lesions of the perineum
    D. cervical hypertrophy   (18:31)

51. Treatment of a teenager on a bad trip includes the following measures, *except*
    A. admitting him to a quiet, nonthreatening environment
    B. physically restraining him to prevent injuring himself and others
    C. establishing verbal contact with reassurance that the experience is temporary and drug related
    D. stressing reality with simple concrete statements regarding his surroundings   (18:37)

52. Large doses of amphetamines may precipitate a hallucinatory state marked by
    A. isolation and depression
    B. euphoria and exhibitionism
    C. grandiosity and feelings of omnipotence
    D. paranoia and aggression (18:37)

53. An important diagnostic sign in barbiturate overdose is
    A. lethargy
    B. hypotension
    C. pinpoint pupils
    D. dilated pupils (18:37)

54. An indicative sign of glutethimide overdose is
    A. lethargy
    B. dilated pupils
    C. hypotension
    D. pinpoint pupils (18:37)

55. The drug that is currently the narcotic antagonist of choice is
    A. naloxone
    B. methadone
    C. nalorphine
    D. levallorphan (18:38)

56. Faliure of naloxone suggests that symptoms are *not* due to overdose of what type of drug?
    A. barbiturate
    B. glutethimide
    C. heroin
    D. opiate (18:38)

57. The abstinence syndrome associated with barbiturate or glutethimide withdrawal is characterized by the following behavioral changes, *except*
    A. apprehension and muscular weakness
    B. postural hypotension
    C. diarrhea
    D. seizure (18:39)

58. Which type of detoxification can be accomplished by the administration of methadone?
    A. opiate
    B. heroin
    C. barbiturate
    D. L.S.D. (18:39)

59. Newborns of addicted mothers usually show the following symptoms, *except*
    A. restlessness, tremors, and convulsions
    B. weakness, vomiting, and diarrhea
    C. high-pitched cry, excessive yawning, and excessive sweating
    D. lethargy, constipation, and hyperpyrexia (18:44)

60. Despite variability from individual to individual, marijuana often causes
    A. temporary impairment of coordination for complex motor activities
    B. distortion of depth and time perception
    C. both A and B
    D. neither A nor B (18:51)

Directions: Match the following numbered items with the most appropriate lettered items.

61. Maintains a 12 hour a day service with clients returning home in evening (18:66)
62. Peer groups discuss their common drug problems and through counseling begin alleviating same (18:66)
63. Serve a full multi-modality programs offering wide range of services (18:66)
64. Man 24 hour telephone service and react to crisis situations in drug-using community (18:65)
65. Motto: "Health is a right, not a privilege." (18:66)

    A. Hotline
    B. Day care centers
    C. Free clinics
    D. Drop-in centers

66. First free clinic on drug abuse (18:70)
67. A 24-hour facility in which patients live in and work in (18:66)
68. In-patient facility for drug abusers (18:69)
69. Establishment oriented (18:70)
70. Therapeutic community (18:66)
71. People-to-people orientation (18:70)

    A. Riverside Hospital, New York City
    B. Haight-Ashbury, San Francisco
    C. Daytop
    D. Youth-type clinic

Social Problems

B 72. Creates relaxation and satisfied well-being (18:80)
C 73. Distorts perception of reality (18:80)
A 74. Gives a feeling of being able to overcome difficulties (18:80)
B 75. Alcohol (18:80)
A 76. Cocaine (18:80)

A. Stimulants
B. Depressants
C. Hallucinogens
D. Emetics

Directions: For each of the following multiple choice questions, select the ONE most appropriate answer.

77. The principle that "Greater satisfaction can be gained in the long run by putting off immediate gratification" is expressed in the
    A. pleasure principle
    B. reality principle
    C. all or none principle
    D. Malthusian principle (18:84)

78. The best means for helping to prevent drug abuse is generally believed to lie in
    A. child's early relationship with the family
    B. inavailability of drugs in local community
    C. formal drug education
    D. peer group influence (18:84)

79. An 18-year-old pregnant female gave birth to a five pound baby boy. She has been addicted to narcotics for 2 years. Her last "fix" was 5 hours before labor and delivery. Which of the following symptoms would *not* be seen in her addicted baby?
    A. diarrhea and vomiting
    B. piercing cry
    C. tremors
    D. lethargy (18:44)

80. Which of the following is *not* a physiological response to amphetamine abuse?
    A. tachycardia
    B. slurred speech
    C. headache
    D. increased perspiration (13:733,734)

81. A sixteen-year-old was struck by an automobile while staggering along the white line in the center of a thoroughfare. Besides those injuries incurred as a result of the accident, the following was noted in the emergency room: chemical smell to breath and reddened and swollen nasopharyngeal mucous membranes which indicate the possible use of
    A. glue
    B. L.S.D.
    C. amphetamines
    D. heroin (13:732)

82. Which of the following is a fallacy about alcoholism?
    A. alcoholism is a progressive and ultimately fatal disease
    B. for alcoholics, alcohol is a drug rather than a beverage
    C. alcoholism can occur only after adult status
    D. alcohol when consumed is absorbed rapidly into the blood stream (13:732)

83. Guidance for therapy of alcoholics of any age may be obtained from
    A. Al-Anon
    B. Alcoholics Anonymous
    C. Synanon
    D. National Council on Alcoholics, Inc. (13:733)

84. Parents can best influence their child against smoking by
    A. absolutely forbidding it
    B. educating him about the harmful effects of smoking
    C. working closely with school
    D. not smoking themselves (13:732)

C. Venereal Diseases

Directions: For each of the following multiple choice questions, select the ONE most appropriate answer.

85. The increase in venereal diseases has been highest in
    A. late childhood
    B. adolescence

C. young adulthood
D. middle age (13:726)

86. The leading cause of death in adolescence is
   A. accidents
   B. drug abuse
   C. malignancy
   D. infections (13:713)

87. In talking with adolescents, the nurse should understand that
   A. nonverbal communication may be as informative as the verbal
   B. if the adolescent immediately begins to talk freely, all formal questions should be withheld
   C. questions should not just be answered, but should be answered by a question put back to them
   D. all of the above (13:696,697)

88. The causative agent of syphilis is a (an)
   A. aerobic bacteria
   B. anaerobic spirochete
   C. virus
   D. aerobic spirochete (10:290)

89. Transmission of Treponema pallidum is primarily by
   A. contact of moist mucous membrane with an infected area
   B. heredity
   C. kissing
   D. contamination with infected needles (10:290)

90. The incubation period of syphilis is about
   A. 7–14 days
   B. 21 days
   C. 10–60 days
   D. 60–120 days (10:291)

91. A standard serologic test for syphilis becomes positive about how soon after infection has been acquired?
   A. 2–3 weeks
   B. 4–5 weeks
   C. 6–7 weeks
   D. 8–9 weeks (10:291)

92. The primary lesion of syphilis is called a (an)
   A. eschar
   B. roseola
   C. chancre
   D. herpes (10:291)

93. Which of the following organs is an unlikely site of the primary lesion of syphilis?
   A. penis
   B. perianal
   C. tongue
   D. ears (10:291)

94. Syphilis is most highly contagious during the
   A. incubation period
   B. primary period
   C. secondary period
   D. late latency stage (10:291)

95. At which stage of syphilis would diagnosis be established only by positive serologic test results?
   A. incubation period
   B. latent or quiescent stage
   C. late latency stage
   D. tertiary stage (10:291)

96. Nervous system involvement or cardiovascular disorders are manifested in what stage of the disease?
   A. primary stage
   B. secondary stage
   C. quiescent stage
   D. late latency stage (10:291)

97. Secondary syphilis may be misinterpreted as the following except
   A. Buerger's disease
   B. acne
   C. impetigo
   D. ringworm (10:291)

98. A drug of choice for syphilis is
   A. cortisone
   B. streptomycin
   C. penicillin
   D. thorazine (10:291)

Social Problems

99. Which of the following is true about syphilis?
    A. effective treatment protects the patient from the disease forever
    B. no relapse and reinfection can very well be differentiated
    C. inadequate doses of antibiotics do not eliminate organisms from lesions tested by means of darkfield examinations
    D. successful treatment yields no immunity to future infection (10:292)

100. The causative agent for gonorrhea is
    A. Neisseria gonorrhoeae
    B. saprophytic neisseria
    C. Neisseria spirochaeta
    D. Neisseria Rickettsia (10:292)

101. The aforenoted causative agent is a
    A. gram-positive intracellular diplococcus
    B. gram-negative intracellular diplococcus
    C. gram-positive extracellular diplococcus
    D. gram-negative extracellular diplococcus

102. Which of the following is *not* true about gonorrhea?
    A. approximately one-third of females infected with the disease will have any symptoms until complications set in
    B. positive smears of vaginal secretions do not necessarily indicate gonorrhea
    C. an adequate serologic test for gonorrhea has not yet been developed
    D. bacteriologic culture procedures demonstrate gonococci in more than 75% of bona fide female contacts (10:292)

103. Gonorrhea in the male is manifested by
    A. purulent urethral discharge three to seven days after sexual contact with an infected partner
    B. purulent urethral discharge a day after sexual contact with an infected partner
    C. generalized lymphadenopathy
    D. hyperpigmented annular lesions (10:292)

104. A common complication of untreated gonorrhea in females is
    A. salpingitis
    B. oophoritis
    C. pelvic inflammatory disease
    D. endocarditis (10:292)

105. Which of the following approaches would be the most important means to prevent the spread of venereal diseases?
    A. forced hospitalization of infected cases
    B. parent education
    C. venereal disease education in schools
    D. V. D. screening of all high school and college students (10:292)

106. Control of venereal disease is a very important aspect of school health. In this area, a school nurse should do the following, *except*
    A. assist other members of school team in case finding
    B. evaluate complaints of students and make necessary referrals to physician
    C. keep adequate health records on all students
    D. prescribe therapy for active cases (13:728)

Directions: Match the following numbered items with the most appropriate lettered items.

107. Local infection of penis (1:171)
108. Pain on urination (1:183)
109. Blood in the urine (13:580)
110. Narrowing of the foreskin tip of the penis (1:171)
111. Meatus is malpositioned dorsally on penile shaft (1:171)
112. Flat, wart-like syphilitic lesion of genital area (1:188)
113. Considered the erectile homologue of the male penis (1:188)
114. Highly infectious, nonsyphilitic genital ulcer (1:188)
115. Absence of menstruation (1:188)
116. Urinary meatus is malpositioned ventrally between glans and scrotum (1:171)

A. Amenorrhea
B. Chancroid
C. Penile hypospadias
D. Dysuria

E. Condyloma latum
F. Balanoposthitis
G. Penile epispadias
H. Vestibule
I. Phimosis
J. Clitoris
K. Chancre
L. Hematuria

D. Juvenile Delinquency

Directions: For each of the following multiple choice questions, select the ONE most appropriate answer.

117. Which of the following is *not* true about the problem of juvenile delinquency?
    A. it refers to acts repeatedly committed by a juvenile which, when committed by adults, are punishable as crimes
    B. it usually includes truancy, running away, incorrigibility and ungovernable behavior
    C. it tends to be self-perpetuating
    D. it is strictly a medical problem (10:272)

118. Most juveniles are referred to court for
    A. running away from home
    B. offenses committed against property
    C. drug peddling
    D. offenses committed against school authorities (10:272)

119. The primary cause of delinquency as shown in extensive studies is
    A. crowded and broken homes
    B. bad companions and less cohesiveness of the family
    C. failure of child to develop strong character and sense of values
    D. all of the above (10:272)

120. Which of the following measures is *least effective* in controlling the problem of juvenile delinquency?
    A. parent education particularly to improve parental responsibility
    B. family neighborhood programs for consciousness raising
    C. institutionalization of all delinquents
    D. counseling to help child cope with his own problem (10:273)

121. The most important aspect of primary prevention of juvenile delinquency is
    A. placing juvenile delinquents in special classes
    B. family counseling services
    C. neighborhood centers for guidance in mental health services
    D. development of a healthy personality of any child (10:273)

122. In helping out the juvenile delinquents, which of these resources might be pooled together for consultation and study of the problem?
    A. family and peer group
    B. teacher and family physician
    C. counselor and policeman
    D. all of the above (10:273,274)

123. Adequate treatment of a delinquent adolescent should have its basic emphasis on the
    A. delinquent act
    B. total individual in his home and community
    C. reasons why he committed such an act
    D. all of the above (13:731)

124. In caring for a delinquent adolescent, it is most important that the nurse basically
    A. accepts him as an individual
    B. makes accurate observation of his behavior
    C. provides him with emotional support
    D. all of the above (13:731)

125. The objectives of juvenile courts are primarily
    A. diagnostic
    B. educational
    C. protective
    D. all of the above (13:731)

Chapter VI: Answers and Explanations

1. **D.**—Child abuse frequently happens in situations where family or financial stress exist and where pent-up frustrations of the parents are focused on the child as a scapegoat.
2. **C.**—It is quite important that Jenny would be able to relate to at least one person in the ward whom she can trust. She needs love and good care.
3. **C.**—Considering Jenny's condition, the picture books would seem to be most appropriate for her. She can derive a lot of enjoyment from looking at the pictures without exerting unnecessary physical energy which may not be advisable for her yet.
4. **C.**—In conjunction with conservation of energy, Jenny should be protected from infections, particularly respiratory infections.
5. **D.**—Indications of congestive heart failure may be a weak cry, cyanotic or pale color, edema, tachycardia and rapid respirations.
6. **D.**—Nursing care must consider the totality of the child.
7. **B.**—The nurse should basically refer the matter to the social service agency. It is generally the responsibility of the physician to report violence against children; however, the nurse should be aware of the policy of the agency and the law of the state in which she is working.
8. **D.**—The nurse should *not* chart her *judgment* that a child had been beaten. She may chart the mother's statements in quotation marks along with the speaker's identity.
9. **C.**—Avoid "empty" calories. Jenny's diet should be planned around the four important food groups.
10. **A.**—Jenny should be exposed to people as much as possible to facilitate socialization. Her care should be built around the general needs of a toddler with due consideration of her special needs.
11. **A.**—Reports have been made that battering parents do not like to be alone as they tend to manifest a lot of anxiety or fears when they are alone.
12. **B.**—Parents subsequently get frustrated and irritated with the child who persistently fails to meet their expectations.
13. **D.**—A nurse who is not resolved about her own feelings concerning a battering parent would not be able to function effectively in caring for a battered child within the context of the family system.
14. **D.**—Management of the parent should be addressed to the totality of his (her) being in relation to the environment rather than to the deviation per se.
15. **B.**—Role reversal, as it applies here, specifically refers to a reversal of the dependency role.
16. **D.**—A broad range of phenomena tends to be reported as child abuse, which may turn out to be erroneous reporting upon investigation.
17. **C.**—Over the years, there have been periodic waves of sympathy and concern from the general public regarding child abuse, rising to a high pitch and then subsiding until the next period of excitation.

18. **D.**—Success of the treatment is reflected in the positive changes seen in the total life of child abusers within the context of man-environment reciprocal relations.
19. **D.**—Child abuse, being a social problem, is best approached within the framework of man-environment reciprocal relations. Therefore, it must necessarily involve all agencies that can contribute to the development of the child and his family.
20. **C.**—The situation implies the availability of at least *one* responsible adult in the family to assume care and custody of the victim.
21. **C.**—The use of heroin could become a consuming preoccupation in the lives of users.
22. **A.**—The hemp plant is scientifically called cannabis sativa.
23. **D.**—Thus the amphetamine user may push himself beyond physical endurance, going without food or sleep for several days.
24. **C.**—Heroin belongs to the family of painkilling drugs derived from opium.
25. **B.**—Although L.S.D. is touted as a "love drug," some people become extremely hostile and suspicious under its influence.
26. **D.**—Extremely heavy amphetamine users may end up psychosis-confused, frightened and out of touch with reality.
27. **C.**—Most young heroin addicts begin by sniffing the substance as early as in elementary school.
28. **B.**—These "flashbacks" may be triggered by bright lights or music or emotional stress.
29. **A.**—Marijuana is related to, but considerably less potent than, hashish.
30. **B.**—The hallucinatory effects are sensory experiences that are not caused by external stimuli.
31. **A.**—Research on the effects of prolonged usage of marijuana has not yet demonstrated significant evidence of physical harm.
32. **C.**—Mescaline comes from the peyote cactus.
33. **A.**—Equanil, a common tranquilizer, acts as a depressant.
34. **C.**—Methedrine is prescribed medically for relief of fatigue, for weight control, and as mood elevators for depressed people.
35. **A.**—Pure L.S.D. is so potent that a tiny drop constitutes a sufficient dose for several users.
36. **D.**—Parents are likely to lose standing with their children when the parents try to act the children's age.
37. **D.**—On the other hand, music can sometimes be "seen" as well as heard by people on an L.S.D. trip.
38. **B.**—The heroin user may go "on the nod," visibly nodding like someone who is half asleep.
39. **D.**—This phenomenon lasts for two or three hours.
40. **A.**—The rush period is readily followed by a period of drowsiness.
41. **C.**—The user is in this condition for two or three hours with corresponding slowing down of physical and mental activities and blurring of reality.
42. **D.**—Parental use of drugs seems to promote children's use of illicit drugs, but this factor has not been cited as a major reason.
43. **A.**—Studies have shown that peer group pressure accounts for over one-half the accountable risk regardless of the drug involved. Low self-esteem is *not* a high risk factor.
44. **D.**—Parental use of drugs *only seems* to promote children's use of drugs.
45. **D.**—The reverse is true. There are far more male drug abusers than female.
46. **B.**—Occlusive thrombophlebitis may be a complication of main lining.
47. **A.**—The heart rate is significantly accelerated and both the systolic and diastolic blood pressure elevated.
48. **C.**—Endocarditis should be suspected in any "mainliner" presenting a fever of unknown origin.
49. **A.**—The aforenoted signs and symptoms are particularly associated with hallucinogenic drugs derived from nutmeg and peyote.
50. **D.**—Cervical erosion and vesicular or ulcerative lesions of the perineum are commonly found among heroin addicted adolescent girls.

51. **B.**—Physical restraint of the patient will almost certainly result in increased anxiety and panic.
52. **D.**—A senile psychotic disorder may follow the termination of amphetamine abuse.
53. **C.**—Pinpoint pupils associated with a history of drug abuse positively indicate barbiturate overdosage.
54. **B.**—Barbiturate and glutethimide overdoses present the same symptoms and signs except for the condition of the pupils.
55. **A.**—Naloxone is preferred to both nalorphine and levallorphan because it does not have respiratory depressant effects; thus, it can be used without risk of accentuating failure if the diagnosis of opiate overdose is erroneous.
56. **A.**—Naloxone is the narcotic antagonist specific for opiate overdose.
57. **C.**—Diarrhea is associated with opiate withdrawal.
58. **A.**—Opiate detoxification does not require hospitalization. It can be accomplished by the administration of methadone, 40 mg. per day gradually reducing the doses over 5 to 10 days.
59. **D.**—When any of the other aforenoted symptoms are seen in the newborn of an addicted mother, the physician generally starts the baby on detoxification treatment.
60. **C.**—Marijuana also causes a transient loss or impairment of memory for recent events.
61. **B.**—Day care centers are hybrid treatment centers which often use modified therapeutic community concepts in the delivery of health care.
62. **D.**—These centers usually deal with multiple drug users and do not get very involved in complicated treatment maneuvers.
63. **B.**—A well run day care center relates to the educational, sexual, psychological, medical and problem solving needs of the young.
64. **A.**—This is probably the simplest and one of the most widely used approaches.
65. **C.**—Free clinics represent a community approach to health care and drug abuse.
66. **B.**—The Haight-Ashbury free clinic for drug abuse was started to provide care and emergency drug abuse intervention.
67. **C.**—In a well run therapeutic community for adolescents, attack and reality therapies are modified, taking into account the fragile egos of young people.
68. **A.**—To many young people, institutions like the Riverside Hospital in New York City represent a barrier to getting help.
69. **D.**—Youth-type clinics are often initiated by service clubs and community organizations.
70. **C.**—Care of the patient should take into account the totality of the man-environment reciprocal relationship.
71. **D.**—Youth-type clinics are examples of free clinics. The concept of "free" simply means no red tape and free of conventional labeling and values.
72. **B.**—Examples of depressants are tranquilizers and barbiturates.
73. **C.**—L.S.D. is a good example of an hallucinogen.
74. **A.**—Amphetamines act as stimulants.
75. **B.**—Alcohol is classified as a depressant.
76. **A.**—Cocaine is a stimulant.
77. **B.**—Drug abusers are usually unable to function according to the reality principle.
78. **A.**—Providing youngsters with a sense of self-esteem during early development, and helping them gain greater confidence through engaging in sustained activities which provide gratification, are likely to keep them away from experimentation with drugs.
79. **D.**—An addicted baby is characteristically restless rather than lethargic.
80. **B.**—Slurred speech is indicative of barbiturate overdosage.
81. **A.**—Adverse effects resulting from glue-sniffing include intense exhilaration, hallucinations, crime and even death.
82. **C.**—Alcoholism is not restricted to any particular age or status. Some alcoholics are alcoholic from their first drink.
83. **B.**—Assistance for members of families of alcoholics may be obtained from Al-Anon.
84. **D.**—Parental influence, especially in the early years of a child's life, is unquestionably strong.
85. **B.**—The incidence is highest among adolescents especially those 15 to 19 years

old. These adolescents are from all socio-economic groups.
86. **A.**—Accidents, specifically motor vehicle accidents, are the principal cause of death. The death rate from illness in this age group is relatively low.
87. **D.**—The nurse must realize that beneath the surface of many routine questions and complaints that young people have, are the real concerns with which they are struggling.
88. **B.**—The organism requires moisture and tissue for survival and dies quickly in the absence of either.
89. **A.**—Transmission by other than human contact with an infected area is most unlikely.
90. **C.**—The incubation period is approximately three weeks, with limits of ten to sixty days.
91. **B.**—Serologic test results are positive in nearly all instances in which secondary lesions have appeared.
92. **C.**—The chancre is of one to five weeks' duration.
93. **D.**—Penile lesions are most frequently found.
94. **C.**—The secondary stage is manifested by a generalized eruption lasting two to six weeks.
95. **B.**—At this time there are no clinical signs or symptoms.
96. **D.**—The late latency stage is otherwise known as the symptomatic period of the disease.
97. **A.**—Other specific skin infections should be ruled out in establishing diagnosis during the secondary stage.
98. **C.**—Inquiry about possible penicillin allergy must always precede such therapy. This is an extremely important precaution.
99. **D.**—It is important to remember that successful treatment of syphilis yields no immunity and there is great difficulty in differentiating between relapse and reinfection.
100. **A.**—To date, no adequate serologic test for gonorrhea has been developed.
101. **A.**—Finding gram-negative intracellular diplococci on smears of vaginal secretions does not necessarily indicate gonorrhea; saprophytic Neisseria species for example will appear identical to Neisseria gonorrhea.
102. **D.**—Studies have shown that bacteriologic culture procedures seldom demonstrate gonococci in more than 50% of bona fide female contacts.
103. **A.**—Symptoms in the acute case may disappear within twenty-four hours of initiation of adequate therapy.
104. **C.**—In most cases, infected females do not show any clinical symptoms until full-blown inflammatory disease develops.
105. **C.**—Preventive education about venereal diseases should be presented to young people at least a year ahead of the time of greatest risk and exposure.
106. **D.**—Prescription of therapy should be under medical direction.
107. **F.**—The condition is characterized by redness and tenderness in both prepuce and glans and sometimes accompanied by discharge.
108. **D.**—Dysuria is oftentimes associated with urgency and frequency.
109. **L.**—Hematuria is a common sign of pathological urinary tract conditions. Hemophilia and leukemia may also be associated with hematuria.
110. **I.**—In older children, a condition called paraphimosis may occur, where the foreskin is permanently retracted behind the corona of the glans and cannot be slipped forward.
111. **G.**—When the meatus is located on the glans, it is called balanic epispadias.
112. **E.**—A wart-like nonsyphilitic projection of the genital area is called condyloma acuminatum.
113. **J.**—The clitoris is an organ composed of erectile tissue which joins the labia minora anteriorly.
114. **B.**—The chancroid should be differentiated from the chancre, a primary syphilitic lesion.
115. **A.**—Amenorrhea can be caused by psychologic factors as well as organic diseases.
116. **C.**—Hypospadias refers to the meatal opening on the ventral surface of the penis.
117. **D.**—Juvenile delinquency goes far beyond the bounds of a medical problem.

Social Problems

118. **B.**—Relatively few commit offenses against a person.
119. **D.**—There is usually a combination of causative factors in any one problem of delinquency.
120. **C.**—Institutionalization of delinquents is hardly an answer to the problem. A combined effort to encourage parental responsibility to improve the neighborhood and develop the child's own resources to cope with his own problems, should be the guiding principle in dealing with juvenile delinquency. Institutionalization should be used sparingly.
121. **D.**—The development of a healthy personality for every child should be the goal of every health worker.
122. **D.**—Any preventive and corrective program must combine the skills of many disciplines to be successful.
123. **D.**—After a study of the total individual, management is planned on the basis of his fundamental problem and what is best for him and for society.
124. **A.**—The nurse must be able to accept him as such without emphasis on his asocial acts.
125. **D.**—The delinquent adolescent can best be managed by personnel in the juvenile courts, instead of the adult courts.